EVERYTHING®
CANDIDA DIET
BOOK

Dear Reader,

Dealing with candida often feels like you are Alice in Wonderland. Realizing that you have candida is like falling into a rabbit hole and emerging into a world where everyone has an opinion, but nothing makes sense.

Fortunately, it doesn't have to be that way. This book is proof that there is a path to understanding candida and a workable approach to controlling it. Over the past thirty years of helping tens of thousands of people overcome candida and restore a foundation of health in their bodies, I've learned that illness is sometimes a gift that points out our weaknesses so we can correct them.

It is said that with great power comes great responsibility. You have a great power within you. In the end, it is your responsibility to heal yourself, and you can!

Jeffrey S. McCombs, DC

Welcome to the EVERYTHING® Series!

These handy, accessible books give you all you need to tackle a difficult project, gain a new hobby, comprehend a fascinating topic, prepare for an exam, or even brush up on something you learned back in school but have since forgotten.

You can choose to read an Everything® book from cover to cover or just pick out the information you want from our four useful boxes: e-questions, e-facts, e-alerts, and e-ssentials.

We give you everything you need to know on the subject, but throw in a lot of fun stuff along the way, too.

We now have more than 400 Everything® books in print, spanning such wide-ranging categories as weddings, pregnancy, cooking, music instruction, foreign language, crafts, pets, New Age, and so much more. When you're done reading them all, you can finally say you know Everything®!

QUESTION

Answers to
common questions

FACT

Important snippets
of information

ALERT

Urgent
warnings

ESSENTIAL

Quick
handy tips

PUBLISHER Karen Cooper

MANAGING EDITOR, EVERYTHING® SERIES Lisa Laing

COPY CHIEF Casey Ebert

ASSISTANT PRODUCTION EDITOR Alex Guarco

ACQUISITIONS EDITOR Eileen Mullan

ASSOCIATE DEVELOPMENT EDITOR Eileen Mullan

EVERYTHING® SERIES COVER DESIGNER Erin Alexander

Visit the entire Everything® series at *www.everything.com*

The
EVERYTHING®
Candida Diet
Book

Improve your immunity by restoring your
body's natural balance

Jeffrey McCombs, DC

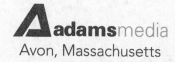

Avon, Massachusetts

To my wife, Ana Maria, and our little angels,
Ana Sophia and Ethan Kai. Love and laughter are the spices
of our lives that make this journey a wonderful gift.

An Everything® Series Book.
Everything® and everything.com® are registered
trademarks of F+W Media, Inc.

Published by
Adams Media, a division of F+W Media, Inc.
57 Littlefield Street, Avon, MA 02322. U.S.A.
www.adamsmedia.com

ISBN 10: 1-4405-7523-1
ISBN 13: 978-1-4405-7523-5
eISBN 10: 1-4405-7524-X
eISBN 13: 978-1-4405-7524-2

Printed in the United States of America.

10 9 8 7 6 5 4 3 2 1

Library of Congress Cataloging-in-Publication Data

McCombs, Jeffrey.
    The everything candida diet book / Jeffrey
McCombs, DC.
        pages cm -- (An everything series book)
Includes index.
ISBN-13: 978-1-4405-7523-5 (pb)
ISBN-10: 1-4405-7523-1 (pb)
ISBN-13: 978-1-4405-7524-2 (ebook)
ISBN-10: 1-4405-7524-X (ebook)
1. Candida--Diet therapy. I. Title.
QK625.C76M33 2014
641.81'5--dc23
                    2014008249

Always follow safety and commonsense cooking
protocol while using kitchen utensils, operating
ovens and stoves, and handling uncooked food. If
children are assisting in the preparation of any recipe, they should always be supervised by an adult.

The information in this book should not be used for
diagnosing or treating any health problem. Not all
diet and exercise plans suit everyone. You should
always consult a trained medical professional
before starting a diet, taking any form of medication, or embarking on any fitness or weight-training
program. The author and publisher disclaim any
liability arising directly or indirectly from the use
of this book.

This book is available at quantity discounts for bulk
purchases.
For information, please call 1-800-289-0963.

Contents

Introduction 9

1 Introduction to Candida 11
What Is Candida? 12
Who Gets Candida? 14
How Does Candida Present Itself? 15
How Long Can Candida Last? 17

2 The Missing Link in Health Care 19
Candida's History 20
The Antibiotic Curse 22
Doctors and Candida 25
Is Candida Dangerous? 27
What Makes Candida Worse? 28

3 Diagnosing Candida 31
How Is Candida Diagnosed? 32
Should You Get Tested? 34
Candida Testing 35
Trusting the Tests 41

4 Treating Candida 45
Medications 46
Herbs 49
Probiotics 56
Fatty Acids 59
What Not to Use to Treat Candida 61

5 Blood-Related Issues Associated with Candida ... 65

Blood Sugar Imbalances 66

Hypoglycemia 66

Hyperglycemia. 69

Diabetes 71

Gestational Diabetes. 72

6 Digestive Problems Associated with Candida. 75

Low Levels of Hydrochloric Acid. 76

Acid Reflux 76

Gastritis 77

Ulcers. 78

Constipation 84

Obesity 85

What about Gluten Intolerance?. 86

7 The Candida Diet 89

The Essentials 90

The Power of Nature. 95

Yes Foods 97

How Long Does It Take? 103

8 Cooking on the Diet. 105

Preparation, Preparation, Preparation 106

Grocery List. 107

Juicing. 108

Spread the Word. 109

Nature's Gifts. 109

Keeping It Simple 110

Dining Out. 111

Genetically Modified Organisms in the Kitchen? 112

9 Breakfast Ideas. 115

10 Appetizers 121

11 Sauces and Marinades 133

12 Salads 151

13 Lunch 157

14 Soups and Stews 165

15 Sides 180

16 Chicken. 217

17 Fish 227

18 Beef and Lamb. 243

19 Beverages. 265

Appendix A: FAQ about Candida 271
Appendix B: Superfoods 281
Standard U.S./Metric Measurement Conversions 293

Index. 294

Acknowledgments

Words can never express my gratitude for the support of my loving wife, Ana Maria. I'm sure that your willingness to support me in all that I do qualifies you for some type of sainthood when all is said and done. Without you, I'd be the only one in the room laughing at my jokes.

To Ana Sophia and Ethan Kai, my one heart became two when you both came along. Each day brings a deeper appreciation of the blessings that you bring to me through your words, gestures, looks, and willingness to take in all that life has to offer. You are the alchemists of my life, transforming nothingness into pure love and joy.

Many thanks to Shannon for your assistance with formatting the recipes, and to Hugo for your wonderful additions to many of the recipes in this book. A big thank-you to Blanca and Hugo for years of willingness to stand beside me in bringing greater health to thousands of lives. Your PhDs are in the mail.

As always, loving thanks to Mom, Kim, Kelly, and Terry, who have always been there. Dad, you are gone, but not forgotten. Look at what you started! Liz, I didn't forget you this time! To J-R and John, my deepest love and gratitude. To all my patients who constantly inspire me to learn more and do better, thank you for the opportunity to serve you.

Thank you to Priscila Satkoff of Salpicón restaurant in Chicago for her amazing recipes in this book.

Lastly, a big thank-you to Adams Media. I needed to quit thinking about all of this stuff and just write it down. You gave me that opportunity. It has helped me to grow and learn even more. Many lives will benefit from this book. Thank you!

Introduction

Candida. Candidiasis. Candida-Related Immune Complex. Systemic Candida. Yeast infection. These terms are all used when discussing candida, an organism that is linked to an increasing amount of diseases and health conditions around the world. You may be familiar with these terms, but if not, eventually you will be. Candida can cause, promote, or contribute to almost any disease or health condition that an individual may experience. From cancer to skin rashes, diabetes to depression, obesity to vaginal infections, candida almost always plays a role. Its effect on the body is widespread, yet its presence is seldom recognized.

The majority of people with systemic fungal candida can go decades without any symptoms, while the slow degeneration of the body's cells and tissues advances. Like most microbes that have existed on this planet for billions of years, candida has developed an amazing ability to adapt instantaneously to all kinds of climates and environments outside of and inside the human body. Yet candida's phantom presence has enabled it to be ignored by modern medicine as a condition worthy of any consideration until it's too late. Abandoned by medicine, even in the face of tens of thousands of studies, candida has been investigated by the scientific community worldwide. Holistic practitioners have rallied to help millions of people looking for an answer that only the recognition and treatment of fungal candida can provide.

Many people are shocked to discover that the mysterious conditions that they've dealt with for years can be so easily explained by candida and its march through their tissues. How can one organism have such a devastating effect on health, yet be unrecognized by the majority of doctors? How can doctors continue to ignore the advances of science in this area while their patients suffer? These questions are not easy to answer.

One possible answer lies with the use of antibiotics. Antibiotics are the class of drugs most prescribed by medical doctors in the world. They are credited with saving millions of lives, they are the backbone of every medical doctor's practice, and they are also the most direct and immediate cause of fungal candida. To the medical profession, antibiotics can do no wrong. Unfortunately, the use of antibiotics creates systemic fungal infections, as well as antibiotic-resistant strains of "superbugs."

Dr. Orian Truss, Dr. William Crook, and Dr. John Trowbridge are among the medical doctors who have led the way in candida research by writing books and papers on the effects of candida in their patients over the past fifty years. Even so, candida is not completely recognized by medical communities.

This book provides time-proven methods for addressing candida. Through the use of a healthful, whole foods–based diet and antifungals, you'll be able to reset your body and improve your health. Leaving behind the Standard American Diet (SAD), which is so commonly associated with heart disease, obesity, diabetes, and a host of other diseases, you'll discover a diet that promotes health, happiness, and longevity. This diet will help reawaken your body's innate ability to regulate itself, and you'll find out which foods provide nourishment and healing. The principles in this book will help you reclaim mastery of your internal landscape. Diet alone won't get you where you need to be, but the diet promoted here can provide a healthful foundation for the rest of your life. A candida diet isn't about restrictions; it's about the freedom that you gain from a life without the symptoms, conditions, and illness associated with today's modern lifestyle and the consequences of unchecked antibiotic use.

Even if you aren't suffering from a condition related to candida, the application of the principles contained in this book can help you reset your body and improve your health.

CHAPTER 1

Introduction to Candida

Some people don't need an introduction to candida; they have been dealing with its effects for years, or even a lifetime. However, starting with the basics will help you better understand what candida is and, sometimes more important, what it is not. Knowing what candida is, where it comes from, who gets it, and how it affects you is the best way to take control of your health and well-being. With this book, you are about to become more knowledgeable about candida than most medical doctors.

What Is Candida?

Is it a yeast or a fungus? Friend or foe? A symbiotic companion or pathogenic intruder? A figment of the imagination or a scientifically valid concern? In reality, candida is all of these, depending on whom you are talking to and the environment that it is found in. Candida can help promote health or contribute to its erosion.

Candida's behavior is primarily governed by the health of a person's intestinal tract and the balance of beneficial bacteria within it, which together form the internal "ecosystem." Anything that alters this ecosystem determines candida's role in the body.

An organism that lives in and on both men and women, candida is one of the many thousands of species of microbes, or "bugs," that call the human body home. Like many of its 100+ trillion cohabitants, candida serves a purpose in the body's internal ecosystem. But unlike many of its fellows, it has a dual nature, existing as either a yeast or a fungus, depending on its environment.

ESSENTIAL

Within a balanced system, both forms of candida can benefit its host. In an imbalanced system, caused by the use of antibiotics, candida rapidly begins to transform from Dr. Jekyll to Mr. Hyde. While the "yeasty" Dr. Jekyll fulfills his role peacefully in a balanced system, the "fungal" Mr. Hyde creates chaos and destruction as he reflects his imbalanced environment.

Yeast to Fungus

The yeasty side of candida ferments sugars and breaks down tissues. While it normally exists in this state, candida can convert to its fungal state given the presence of appropriate triggers, such as pH, temperature, sugars, certain compounds, and a lack of bacteria to prevent its growth. Although a weakened immune system is another trigger, it is less instrumental in the initial transformation. However, the use of antibiotics alone can cause all of these triggers to present at once. Other factors like hormones and toxins may cause one trigger to become active, but that alone will not cause the transformation.

Once the transformation has taken place and the fungal monster appears, candida quickly leaves the intestinal tract and enters the bloodstream. The strong presence of immune cells in the blood prevents candida from spending much time there, so it rapidly enters all the tissues of the body, where it starts to secrete enzymes, break down the tissues, and derive nutrients.

When viewing candida under a microscope, candida's yeast form looks like a single round cell, while as a fungus, it has a branchlike formation that grows and intertwines, much like a tumbleweed. This appearance can make candida look like a tumor when seen on an x-ray. The fungal form has enhanced abilities as well; for example, research has shown that candida can manipulate the immune system to favor the organism's growth. In addition to its enzymes, candida promotes the production of other strong inflammatory enzymes within the body. It becomes a vicious cycle: Inflammation promotes the growth of candida and candida promotes inflammation. As candida grows and spreads in the absence of the bacteria that normally inhibit its growth, it also helps dictate which bacteria will grow back after having been eliminated by antibiotics. This process, which can occur in only a few days, can create a lifelong imbalance.

Friend or Foe

It is possible that candida's fungal form could also be beneficial. In a balanced system, the body could help create the yeast-to-fungus conversion so the fungal form uses its enzymes to break down dead and decaying matter, which is one of the main roles of fungus on this planet. Although candida has been identified as a cause of cancer, others researchers have noted that the presence of candida at the site of a cancerous tumor assists in breaking down the tumor, rather than causing it.

It makes sense that both the yeast and fungal forms can play beneficial roles. Were it not for the widespread devastation that antibiotic use causes in the body's internal ecosystem, the fungal candida problem may never have surfaced to such a degree. Life without candida and its pathogenic, problematic side would have been the norm.

A Figment of Your Imagination

It is not easy to dismiss the rapidly growing number of people who are afflicted with candida and the staggering body of associated research. Candida has become the number-one fungal infection and fourth leading cause of infectious deaths in hospitals. More and more people are realizing that many of their symptoms are due to candida. It may well be that a grassroots awareness of candida moves this orphaned condition into the forefront of medicine.

Who Gets Candida?

Most men who have heard of candida think that only women can be affected by it. This is a grand misconception. Candida resides in men, women, and children. The misperception that candida exists only in those people with suppressed immune systems has now been corrected by scientists worldwide. Not only was fungal candida found in people with AIDS and cancer, but also in patients with diabetes and in patients who are hospitalized for any reason. Individuals with nutritional deficiencies and alcoholism are excellent candidates. Even people with no problems at all are susceptible to fungal candida infections.

As science has shown, antibiotic use appears to be the leading cause of fungal candida infections today. Given that most people have been exposed to antibiotics several times, it is likely that just as many people have fungal candida growth. Once antibiotics have been taken, only twenty-four to forty-eight hours are needed for fungal candida to pass through the intestinal wall and enter the bloodstream. One study detailed on *www.nih.gov* showed that fungal growth in the kidneys twenty-four hours after candida entered the bloodstream. So far, antibiotics appear to be a two-edged sword. Other medications like steroids and birth-control pills have also been linked to fungal candida, but they don't create the same effects as antibiotics. Although these medications may contribute to conditions that favor fungal overgrowth, they are less likely, in and of themselves, to be the cause.

QUESTION

What if I have many of the symptoms of candida, but have never taken antibiotics?
Today, it seems almost impossible not to experience an ongoing exposure to antibiotics in foods and liquids. Consider antibacterial soaps, for example. Small exposures accumulate over time and have lasting effects. A poor diet combined with stress and exposure to chemicals and heavy metals can impact the body as well.

How Does Candida Present Itself?

Considering all of the conditions and symptoms reportedly linked to a candida infection, the "everything" adjective in the title of this book seems appropriate. Candida has been associated with more than 100 symptoms and conditions, ranging from simple gas and bloating to complex autoimmune conditions, like diabetes and lupus.

Inflammation

Inflammation is the link between candida and many of the conditions and symptoms that it is believed to contribute to. Candida is a very strong promoter of inflammation, since inflammation helps advance its growth. Inflammation is also part of the immune response to promote healing. The process by which the immune system responds to candida's presence in the tissues and fluids helps create the ideal conditions for it to thrive and wreak havoc. Researchers like Dr. Christina Zielinski, at the Institute for Research in Biomedicine, have helped identify this phenomenon in greater detail. Dr. Zielinski and her team have detailed the steps the immune system takes to produce an inflammatory response to candida's presence. She links this response to autoimmune diseases like rheumatism, psoriasis, and Crohn's disease.

The same immune cells noted by Zielinski have also been implicated in multiple sclerosis, diabetes, lupus, allergies, and asthma. These immune cells can help create a healing response over the short term, but their prolonged presence also helps create chronic inflammation and tissue damage. Another team of researchers from the University of California at San

Diego has shown that a class of enzymes, like those produced by candida, can cause hypertension, diabetes, and immune system suppression. Science continues to amass a significant amount of data on the many ways in which candida affects the body.

Candida is believed to be associated with conditions such as:

- Acid reflux
- Acne
- ADD, ADHD
- Allergies
- Anxiety
- Arthritis
- Asthma
- Athlete's foot
- Autism
- Autoimmune conditions
- Benign prostatic hypertrophy
- Bladder infections
- Blisters in the mouth
- Bloating
- Blood sugar imbalances
- Body odor
- Brain fog
- Bronchitis
- Burping
- Cancer
- Chemical sensitivities
- Chronic fatigue syndrome
- Colitis
- Concentration problems
- Confusion
- Congestion
- Constipation
- Cough
- Crohn's disease
- Cystitis
- Depression
- Dermatitis
- Diabetes
- Diarrhea
- Eczema
- Endometriosis
- Excess mucus
- Fibromyalgia
- Flatulence
- Fluid retention
- Food allergies
- Food cravings
- Frequent colds
- Frequent infections
- Fungal infections
- Gas
- Gastritis
- Genital rashes
- Gluten allergy
- Headaches
- Heartburn
- Hormonal imbalances
- Hypoglycemia
- Hypothyroidism
- Irritability
- Inflammatory bowel disease
- Immune system dysfunction
- Impotence
- Indigestion
- Infertility
- Irregular menstruation
- Itchy skin

- Joint pain
- Lack of mental clarity
- Leaky gut (increased permeability of the intestinal wall)
- Lethargy
- Lupus
- Memory problems
- Meningitis
- Migraines
- Mood swings
- Multiple sclerosis
- Muscle spasms
- Nail fungus
- Osteoarthritis
- Penile itching
- PMS
- Poor memory
- Prostatitis
- Psoriasis
- Rashes
- Rectal itching
- Rheumatoid arthritis
- Rhinitis
- Scleroderma
- Sinus problems
- Sores
- Sore throat
- Sugar cravings
- Swollen joints
- Thrush
- Ulcers
- Urethritis
- Urinary frequency
- Vaginal infections
- Vaginitis
- Visual problems
- Weakness
- Weight gain
- White coating on tongue

If you don't find your symptoms on this list, you may not have a fungal candida problem. Some people attribute everything they are experiencing to candida, which can delay finding the proper answer. If you don't have any of these symptoms, but you've taken antibiotics, bear in mind that one hospital study titled "Symptomatic and asymptomatic candidiasis in a pediatric intensive care unit" showed that the majority of people who had candida had no symptoms. Undergoing testing for candida can provide more answers, and talking with a knowledgeable health-care practitioner can be invaluable.

How Long Can Candida Last?

The greater the diversity of any ecosystem, the greater its health will be. This is true for ecosystems around the world, as well as the one in your gut. Once an ecosystem is altered, its health will change according to the alteration. Antibiotics reduce the diversity of the gut each and every time they are used. This also occurs when antibiotics are dumped into ecosystems around the world, leading to permanent shifts in the resident microbes, plants, fish, and animal species. Multiple rounds of antibiotics can greatly reduce the diversity of the gut's microbial populations. In their wake, antibiotics leave an imbalanced system filled with antibiotic-resistant strains of bacteria and fungal candida. Science has shown that this change is permanent and can shape our health for years to come.

FACT

In 2003, in an effort to minimize the risks inherent in antibiotic use, the FDA mandated that all doctors first isolate bacterial infections and then test for their susceptibility to available antibiotics before writing a prescription. Although this is a federal mandate, a law intended to protect Americans, medical doctors rarely comply.

From a clinical perspective, it is common to find people who can relate their health issues to taking antibiotics. As bacteria are eliminated and fungal candida grows, the candida overgrowth will prevent the return of certain bacteria, mainly the *Lactobacillus* genus. This alteration has been associated with nutrient deficiencies and conditions like gastritis, ulcers, gas, bloating, indigestion, allergies, and sinus problems.

However, since most people with systemic candida are asymptomatic, relying on symptoms as an indicator of health can be misleading. The body has a great ability to adapt. This adaptation can make life easier, but it can mask problems that have been brewing for years. Cause and effect is a poor model in health care; sometimes it can take a lifetime for diseases and conditions to appear, which makes the accurate identification of causes problematic.

Candida drives chronic inflammation, and the change that inflammation creates is one of the main factors in all diseases. Given that antibiotics create permanent alterations to the microbial flora and that fungal candida is a part of those changes, it is likely that fungal candida can last a lifetime unless specific steps are taken to restore the normal bacterial flora and transform candida to its normal yeast form. This book gives you the tools to identify, test for, and safely correct the effects of candida. With the right tools and the opportunity to change, you can create a healthy mind and body.

CHAPTER 2

The Missing Link
in Health Care

Over the past sixty years, a widening gap has occurred between science and the current practice of medicine. Unfortunately, undiagnosed candida falls into this gap. Millions of patients suffer from its effects, yet very few doctors know anything about it even though tens of thousands of scientific studies have documented the condition.

Candida's History

Candida, as it is known today, is a relatively new concern in health care. Its historical record, however, dates back to the fifth century B.C. when the Greek physician Hippocrates described white oral plaques on the tongue and mouth of his patients. Over the next two thousand years, the condition had various names until Christine Berkhout described the genus as *Candida* in 1923. Still considered a relatively rare condition until the introduction of antibiotics in 1944, candida's subsequent rise in popularity and occurrence paralleled the increased usage of antibiotics from 1944 to the present. According to the National Institutes of Health's National Library of Medicine, there were no studies recorded on candida in 1944. The following year there were five studies, and since then, more than fifty-two thousand studies have been added to the database; approximately seven new studies are added every day.

FACT

The Greek physician Hippocrates (460–370 B.C.) is revered as the Father of Medicine. The Hippocratic oath taken by all doctors pays homage to his philosophy and views.

First Cases

Some of the first cases of fungal candida in humans diagnosed after the introduction of antibiotics involved skin conditions like psoriasis. People who had no prior history of dermatological issues before taking antibiotics were developing severe cases that required medical attention and care. Doctors noted that most, if not all, of these new cases occurred following the use of the new antibiotic therapies. Early treatments consisted of high doses of undecenoic acid prescribed topically and internally. The cure rates were impressive, but the treatment fell out of use when antifungal drugs were developed.

Candida albicans

Scientists have discovered from 150 to 350 species of candida, depending on the source cited. Of these, only a few are known to cause diseases.

The most common form to affect humans is *Candida albicans*. It has historically been known more for the oral thrush form and the vaginal form. Scientists have found that other forms like *Candida dubliniensis, C. parapsilosis, C. glabrata, C. krusei,* and *C. tropicalis* are occurring more frequently, but still lag far behind *C. albicans*. Even when another form is found, *C. albicans* will almost always be present as well.

Polymorph

Although candida normally occurs in its yeast form in the body, scientists have been unraveling the many mechanisms by which it converts to its fungal form and then begins to spread. Candida has been described as a polymorph or dimorphic organism due to its ability to convert from one form to another. To date, pH, temperature, availability of food, bacteria, and cells of the immune system have been listed as factors controlling the organism's ability to transform. Of these, pH and the presence or absence of other bacteria in the area tend to be the most important factors controlling the conversion.

Virulence

Once the transformation takes place, there is little stopping candida from becoming systemic. The yeast-to-fungal transformation takes from one to six hours. Once converted, candida quickly crosses the intestinal wall and starts to cause tissue damage within twenty-four to forty-eight hours by employing an array of enzymes that can break down the protein, fat, and carbohydrate layers of cells and tissues that might oppose its intrusion. Candida's ability to adapt is almost instantaneous. Not only can it survive attacks from the immune system, it can manipulate immune responses and destroy immune cells. Along with its own enzymes, candida increases other enzymes within the body that are known to play a role in the breakdown of tissues.

QUESTION

Does candida affect pets as well?
Yes, candida affects animals and humans alike, although less research has been done on animals. Therapies that are successful in treating pets are those also used in humans.

The Antibiotic Curse

The development of antibiotic-resistant strains of bacteria has rendered many antibiotics useless for increasing numbers of people. Very few new antibiotics are being developed. With no hope of profiting from the development of antibiotics, pharmaceutical companies are investing time and money in other classes of drugs.

The Human Paradox

Beneath the antibiotic-resistance debate lies an often-overlooked problem with the use of all antibiotics. Perhaps nothing points to this paradox more clearly than the meaning of the word *antibiotic*: "against life." Life is based on the extremely complex, yet delicate interaction of 10 trillion human cells with the 100 trillion cells of the micro-organisms that fill, cover, and line every inch of the body.

Humans and the microbes that accompany them are no longer viewed as separate organisms coexisting in the same space but as one superorganism. Anything that affects the health of one affects the health of the other. In addition to these microbes being responsible for developing the immune system, synthesizing nutrients, protecting the body from toxic chemicals and radiation, and keeping out pathogenic organisms that cause disease, they also help maintain the genetic pool and the development of the infant's brain. Some studies even suggest that these microbes play a role in fertility.

Antibiotics, unfortunately, can be detrimental to the microbes. A five- to seven-day course of antibiotics can wipe out all the bacteria in the body. It takes these bacteria nine to twelve months to repopulate, and some never return. As a result, antibiotics create a permanent alteration of the gut bacteria and of the health of the body.

The Hidden Epidemic

Antibiotics are used as though they can target a select group of organisms and leave the rest alone. On the contrary, acting more like a nuclear weapon, antibiotics destroy everything within reach, leaving a desolate, barren landscape open to colonization by the bacteria that respond most quickly. The logical first responders will be bacteria and microbes that are not affected by antibiotics, such as yeast, parasites, mold, and viruses.

Candida has always been one of the fastest responders. In the absence of 100 trillion opposing bacterial cells, candida rapidly converts from yeast to fungus, escapes its confinement in the intestinal tract, and quickly spreads via the circulatory system. Without the normal system of checks and balances in place, candida quietly establishes itself throughout the body, using its enzymes to obtain nutrients from the surrounding cells and tissues.

Antibiotics seem to create every condition necessary for candida's transformation. While other drugs may enable one or two of these conditions, antibiotics provide them all. Here are at least ten known methods by which antibiotics enable candida's transformation:

- By destroying bacteria that inhibit the growth and conversion of candida
- By destroying bacteria that secrete lactic acids known to keep candida in its yeast form
- By destroying bacteria that secrete fatty acids, such as butyric acid, known to inhibit candida
- By causing the release of intracellular components in bacteria that trigger the conversion
- By suppressing white blood cells, like macrophages, that inhibit candida
- By suppressing chemical messengers (chemokines) that alert immune cells to candida's presence
- By suppressing chemical messengers (cytokines) that hide iron from candida and other microbes that need it for their growth
- By destroying bacteria that synthesize the B vitamins necessary for production of stomach acid that inhibits candida's conversion
- By causing a massive release of substances that damage the intestinal cells and facilitate candida's escaping confinement in the intestinal tract
- By directly causing candida to convert

As science learns more about how candida and other microbes function in the presence of antibiotics, this list will continue to grow. Antibiotics create a perfect storm for the conversion of this normally beneficial yeast to a problematic, pathogenic fungal organism. From acne to cancer, the possible effects of fungal candida are numerous.

The Antibiotic Myth

The myth: Antibiotics are prescribed by medical doctors, who represent the pinnacle of modern medical care; therefore, antibiotics must be good, otherwise, doctors wouldn't prescribe them. That seems a fair enough assumption, but it leads to the further supposition that antibiotics are harmless—and that belief is inaccurate and potentially dangerous.

Antibiotics have been linked to increased risk of breast and colon cancer; kidney, lung, and nerve damage; lupus; asthma; arthritis; liver failure; strep throat; pancreatitis; obesity; diabetes; allergies; nutrient deficiencies; sudden death; immune system suppression; and increased susceptibility to infections. The list of side effects is much longer. Prescribed primarily for infections, antibiotics can actually suppress the immune system and increase the risk of getting more infections. Does it make sense to suppress the immune system when there is an infection? Isn't the infection proof that the immune system is already suppressed? Candida wastes no time in taking advantage of this situation to establish itself.

QUESTION

I've taken antibiotics, and I've felt better. Isn't this proof that they helped me?
Antibiotics suppress the immune system's healing response, which promotes inflammation and creates fevers, aches, pains, and that overall feeling of sickness. Although eliminating these symptoms can make you feel better, antibiotics can interfere with the body's immune system and leave you more vulnerable to additional infections.

Always consider the risks when taking antibiotics. They are never risk-free and are frequently overprescribed. The end result of taking antibiotics is fungal candida. If you need to take antibiotics, consider taking probiotics as well. After your course is finished, you'll need to address fungal candida and a multitude of other possible long-term effects.

Doctors and Candida

Some doctors, though not all, believe that candida is a valid concern only when there is a systemic blood infection in an immunosuppressed patient. But researchers from the University of Cincinnati have revealed that "candida is the leading cause of invasive fungal disease in premature infants, diabetics, and surgical patients." Researchers from the Whitehead Institute for Biomedical Research have stated that "candida is also a major cause of infection in hospitalized patients, especially those in Intensive Care Units, patients after major injuries or surgery, patients with burns, and premature babies." Researchers from the Washington Hospital Center and the Boston University School of Medicine have added the elderly, those with nutritional deficiencies, and patients with anything that penetrates the skin (catheters, IV lines, feeding tubes) to the list of those susceptible to candida. Researchers from the Royal Postgraduate Medical School of London and Westminster Hospital have stated that there is no common "immunological denominator" to account for candida.

ALERT

Individuals who are being treated with chemotherapy, immunosuppressant drugs, or HIV medications should discuss possible options for prevention and treatment of systemic fungal candida infections. The chance for blood-borne candida infections and fatalities is highest in this group.

One of the most prominent researchers on candida, Jean-Marcel Senet from the Laboratory of Immunology, Parasitology, and Mycology in Angers, France, states that candida infections can follow "even very slight environmental modifications" of the host. Researchers from Louisiana State University Medical Center and BIOCODEX pharmaceutical, Montrouge,

France, have strayed the farthest from medical opinion by showing that candida spreads in individuals who have no immune system suppression or weakness.

FACT

Sally Davies, chief medical officer for the United Kingdom, has assessed the growing epidemic of antibiotic-resistant "superbugs" worldwide and stated that "antimicrobial resistance poses a catastrophic threat" to all humans. Even Alexander Fleming, who discovered penicillin, noted that bacteria were quick to develop resistance to penicillin.

Many researchers commonly implicate antibiotics as the main cause of candida. Stone and colleagues, from Emory University School of Medicine, state that "oral antibiotic therapy in humans often leads to colonization and over-growth of the GI tract by *C. albicans*," and Seelig, MD, states that " . . . the preponderance of evidence indicates that the use of antibiotics is associated with an increased incidence of candidiasis and fungal infections." You can read the full study at *www.ncbi.nlm.nih.gov*.

These few examples are a sampling of the thousands of scientific papers that clearly demonstrate and clarify the effects of candida and antibiotics.

ESSENTIAL

To find an alternative medical doctor who has received training in alternative medical practices, contact either the American Holistic Medical Association (*www.holisticmedicine.org*) or the American Board of Integrative Holistic Medicine (*www.abihm.org*).

Should you choose to see a medical doctor for candida, remember that candida might be an unknown to them. Risk-benefit analysis applies as much to seeing a medical doctor as it does to taking a drug. Only you can decide if it's worth it. More and more people who have slipped through the gaps of medical knowledge seek compassionate, reliable care elsewhere with alternative medical practitioners. It's an option worth considering.

Is Candida Dangerous?

This question could apply to almost any condition. To give an accurate answer, it is important to assess the overall health of the patient. Is he young or old? Does he take medications; if so, which medications and how long has he been taking them? Has he had surgery recently? What other conditions does he have? What is his family health history? What's his diet like?

The Suppressed Immune System

In an individual with an extremely suppressed immune system, candida ranks as the fourth-leading cause of death in hospitals as an infectious agent, and the number-one killer among fungal infections. These patients generally have AIDS or cancer, or are receiving immunosuppressant drugs in cases of organ transplants and certain autoimmune diseases. Obviously, in this group of people, candida is very dangerous, racing throughout the bloodstream, unchecked by their immune system and other defenses. Treatment involves powerful antifungal drugs that unfortunately cause further suppression of the immune system. Under these circumstances, fewer than 50 percent of these patients survive.

QUESTION

How can I determine how strong my immune system is?
Lymphocyte Subset Panels are blood tests that evaluate the activity of immune cells in the body. These comprehensive immune panels tend to be costly and are offered by very few laboratories. Testing for the presence of chemicals and heavy metals can help establish a better assessment of overall health.

Certain levels of immunosuppression due to accumulating levels of chemicals and heavy metals, as well as the immune-depleting effects of stress and poor dietary habits, allow the spread of candida but are not enough to enable it to become life-threatening. Older individuals tend to have weaker immune systems and may exhibit more complications, or they may have no symptoms at all.

Cancer

Cancer, in general, takes years, decades, and sometimes a lifetime to develop. Most toxins do not produce noticeable effects until they have created enough damage or change to the body's genetic blueprint or defenses that it starts producing the abnormal cells and tissues identified as cancerous. This process requires the toxin to work consistently on the body. Candida is very efficient here since it creates the strongest element associated with all cancer: chronic inflammation.

Chronic inflammation tears down, wears down, and damages the cells, tissues, DNA, and the body's defenses; causes rapid aging; and can lead to all types of cancer. Fungal candida drives inflammation, which in turn promotes the growth and spread of the fungus. It is the mechanism by which candida can play a role in many conditions. Candida can also alter and suppress the immune responses that help prevent cancer. Although it is not immediately threatening in these cases, candida's potential effect over the long term adds to the inherent danger present.

What Makes Candida Worse?

While antibiotics lay the foundation for the establishment of fungal candida throughout the body, other factors can play a role in fueling its existence, suppressing its restraints, or modifying its effects. The main coconspirators include diet, medications, stress, and other infections.

Diet

The Standard American Diet, whose unfortunate but very telling acronym is SAD, is a precursor to many diseases and conditions. Some societies around the world that have adopted this diet has witnessed an increase in obesity, diabetes, and heart disease. This type of diet is high in sugars and in processed foods, which include lots of simple carbohydrates that rapidly break down into sugars. Sugars and simple carbohydrates support the overgrowth of fungal candida. A diet that is high in sugars will effectively fuel candida's growth. It will also suppress the immune system and remove some of the restraints that an active immune system provides against candida.

Removing food sources of sugars and simple carbs can help limit the overgrowth of candida.

Medications

Other than antibiotics, steroids, birth control pills, and chemotherapy have also been associated with candida overgrowth. Steroids and chemotherapy can cause suppression of an immune system that restrains and helps contain candida. Chemotherapy, like antibiotics, can also create all the factors necessary for the organism's rapid growth and spread. Unlike antibiotics, however, chemotherapy is not commonly used and therefore is less associated with the fungal overgrowth found in most people. Birth control pills contain hormones that help facilitate its growth. While they can't produce the effects associated with antibiotics, birth control pills can help promote and maintain its presence.

Stress

Stress is often defined as the basis for all diseases. It affects the intricate machinery of the cells and the major functions of the organs. Like candida, stress can suppress the immune system, affect blood sugar levels, disrupt hormones, alter brain function, and drive inflammation. The chaos of today's world is a state that no one is well equipped to handle. Reducing the effects of both candida and stress can go a long way toward creating a healthier life.

Other Pathogens

As if creating the ideal conditions for candida wasn't enough, antibiotics also create antibiotic-resistant strains of bacteria that are known to help protect and facilitate the growth of fungal candida. Many advanced pathogenic organisms, like *E. coli* and salmonella, have been shown to enable candida's growth. Some pathogens alter immune responses and the bacterial environment, and others actually form a protective layer, or biofilm, over candida to protect it. Since they are also resistant to antibiotics, these superbugs occupy the body's immune responses, which provides time for candida to flourish.

FACT

In 2011, antibiotic-resistant *Clostridium difficile* infections surpassed *E. coli* as the number-one cause of infectious deaths in the United States. A report by *USA Today* estimates that approximately 30,000 deaths occur each year in the United States due to *C. difficile*. Antibiotic-resistant strains of *Staphylococcus aureus* kill an additional 19,000 Americans each year.

CHAPTER 3

Diagnosing Candida

Once an individual discovers that candida can explain many, if not all, of the symptoms that he has been experiencing, he will start to look for some type of confirmation. A doctor or therapist who is knowledgeable about candida, what creates it, and how it functions in the body should be able to provide assistance without the need for testing. However, there are several ways to reveal the presence of candida in the body.

How Is Candida Diagnosed?

Candida is often best diagnosed based on past health history, signs and symptoms, history of antibiotic use, and the results of following any type of antifungal diet. Laboratory testing is another choice. All of this information can provide the best clinical picture for determining whether there is a candida imbalance in the body.

ESSENTIAL

Dr. Arturo Casadevall of Albert Einstein College of Medicine explains balance in the body: ". . . there are only microbes and hosts and the outcomes of their interactions, which include commensalism, colonization, latency, and disease." Stated another way, balance in the body is not just dependent on whether you are exposed to an infectious bug, it's about your body's state of health and how your body responds.

Past Health

Each person's health history will play a role in his future state of health. Current scientific literature states that the health of an individual's great-grandparents is also a factor in being able to predict that person's health. To accurately determine the impact of a patient's health history, therefore, a doctor would need to examine several generations of the person's family.

Your health history can provide many clues to your current health. If you have frequent colds and infections, your immune system is likely having difficulty regulating the 100 trillion microbes that live in and on the body. The use of medications can also suppress immune function or alter the ability to process foods, regulate hormones, control inflammation, eliminate toxins, or any number of bodily processes.

A diet high in sugars and processed fats and carbohydrates can lead to obesity, diabetes, and other metabolic diseases. Certain races are more predisposed to certain conditions. Where you live and where you grew up are additional factors. Past surgeries and a stressful lifestyle are also major factors. All of these elements play a role in establishing and maintaining fungal candida.

Signs and Symptoms

As discussed in Chapter 1, the list of signs and symptoms believed to be associated with candida numbers well over 100 strong and is still growing. The more common ones include indigestion, gas, bloating, skin rashes, acne, constipation, brain fog, allergies, arthritis, sinus problems, blood sugar and hormonal imbalances, vaginal infections, weight gain, gastritis, and acid reflux. Anything associated with inflammation, as most signs and symptoms are, can be related to candida. The longer you've had candida, the more chronic the inflammation, and the more likely it is that you will have candida. Be sure to look at current signs and symptoms, as well as past ones. Any active phase of fungal candida growth may produce symptoms that fade as it becomes more established and the body adapts to its presence. Symptoms are based on feedback loops in the body.

FACT

A feedback loop is created when the body's sense organs, such as nerve cells, relay information to the brain, spinal cord, or other nerve cells to help generate awareness on some level of the external or internal environment. This feedback then allows the body to respond in an appropriate way.

Feedback loops can break down and stop functioning for various reasons such as degeneration, loss of nutrients, adaptation, or genetic changes. Candida itself may induce changes in cells, including immune responses, that alter their ability to respond appropriately.

ESSENTIAL

Micro-organisms have 360 microbial genes for each human gene. In the human body, there are ten microbe cells for every human cell.

Antifungal Diet

How your body reacts to an antifungal diet can also help establish a diagnosis. Candida thrives on sugars and simple carbohydrates. Cutting out sugars, cakes, cookies, breads, pasta, chips, crackers, fruit juices, dried fruit, colas, and most grains can improve anyone's health for many reasons, including fungal candida.

Earlier recommendations of foods to avoid on an antifungal diet included all fruits and starchy vegetables, like potatoes, sweet potatoes, and yams, but recent studies have shown that the body requires some carbohydrates for normal function. Candida diets that are based on a scientific approach generally include most fruits and starchy vegetables. If you have blood sugar issues, you may have to avoid these initially as well.

If your symptoms improve when following this type of diet, you may have an overgrowth of fungal candida. If you need to eliminate all fruits and starchy vegetables to feel some improvement, you may have a problem regulating your blood sugar levels. Candida has been linked to blood sugar imbalances and even diabetes, but you should also consider chemicals, heavy metals, and stress.

Should You Get Tested?

When faced with the complexities surrounding most conditions, having the "cold, hard facts" might be the easiest way to assess an imbalance. Most people see standard laboratory testing as a reliable way to evaluate the presence of candida.

QUESTION

Do I need to see a physician to get tested?
Most tests will require some interaction with a doctor, whether conducted through an office visit, telephone conversation, e-mail, or website. The doctor is the point person for the laboratories' communications. Most of the time, a test kit will be sent to the patient to collect a sample at home.

Testing takes several forms, including blood, stool, urine, saliva, and direct-tissue tests. Direct-tissue testing is the most reliable, because it requires less interpretation. It is also the least-used test since it is invasive, involving a biopsy or collection of body fluids. This form of testing can be used with vaginal surfaces, skin lesions, and oral conditions where the tissues or fluids are more easily accessible.

For a systemic infection, blood, stool, and urine tests are more frequently used. If you have a history of antibiotic use and have symptoms that are commonly associated with candida, then testing can be an excellent way to assess the presence of fungal candida. If you have followed a candida diet and benefited from it, that can be further confirmation. It is best to be tested before and after a candida diet and using any type of fatty acid, herb, or medication. Notice if your symptoms have resolved. Unresolved symptoms can indicate an unsuccessful treatment approach or an additional cause of the symptoms that commonly includes heavy metals, chemicals, and stress. Learning to monitor your body's responses to your internal and external environment is a good practice to incorporate into your daily life. Your body is giving you feedback for a reason. Learn to listen to it!

Candida Testing

As technology advances, there are greater improvements that more quickly and accurately identify the presence of fungal candida. Direct-tissue and fluid sampling is the most accurate test available, but it is limited to just a few conditions such as oral, vaginal, and skin infections. Using a combination of tests can create a better picture of what's taking place deeper within the body. Becoming familiar with the available options can help you and your doctor determine which tests would serve you best.

ALERT

People who have difficulty with blood tests should use either the stool or urine tests. Blood samples must be drawn at a lab.

Testing for candida via blood, stool, and urinary markers can also be combined with additional tests that may highlight imbalances in the intestinal flora and function. Such tests look at hydrochloric acid levels in the stomach, or for the presence of parasites. The only limit in utilizing a combination of tests will usually be financial constraints.

Stool Tests

Collected in the privacy of your home, the sample is mailed to the lab in envelopes provided with the test kits. The results, along with the laboratory's interpretation, are sent to the doctor who can explain and interpret them for you. No needles are involved and no doctor visit is required in most cases.

The collection instructions are similar for each lab. Examining the stool allows a doctor to view the composition and function of the intestinal tract, which includes the bacteria, yeasts, and fungi, as well as fatty acids, pH, red blood cells, dietary fibers, and enzymes. Some labs also analyze any parasites found. The presence or absence of each element helps determine the health of the digestive tract. Each lab examines the samples microscopically and uses other instrumentation that might include gas chromatography to determine the constituents of the stool. Gas chromatography is a process in which the stool is mixed with a liquid and then vaporized within a tube. Instruments measure the chemical compounds present in the vapor. The average stool is estimated to be about 30 percent bacteria by weight. A comprehensive stool analysis will try to determine whether candida, or any beneficial or harmful bacteria or parasites, are present. The number of species investigated varies from lab to lab. Additional information can include markers for inflammation, immune function, enzymatic function, and digestion.

To avoid affecting the results of the tests, you will usually have to stop taking antifungals, antibiotics, and probiotics at least two weeks prior to collecting the samples. Two to three days before, you may also be asked to avoid enzymes, clay powders, and anti-inflammatory drugs such as aspirin and ibuprofen. You will be encouraged to follow your typical diet since this determines to a great degree the current and recent composition of the bacteria in the intestinal tract. Some labs may ask you to increase your fat consumption to measure how well you handle fats. If you have a severe infection of the intestinal tract, you may be asked to wait until the infection resolves. In this case, it is probably best to consult with your doctor to determine when to collect the samples.

Depending on the laboratory, there are two main approaches to collecting and analyzing the stool samples. The first approach, which is the oldest and most common, is to collect three samples and send them to the lab. The overall findings are then averaged among the three samples. One advantage is that three samples may catch daily variations found in the stool that a single specimen might miss. In the second approach, you collect only one sample. The stool is placed in a tube containing a solution that, in effect, "freezes" it, thus preventing the rapid die-off and loss of microbes that occur from exposure to oxygen.

This approach uses a polymerase chain reaction (PCR), which looks for the DNA or genetic pieces of a microbe. This is about as small a sampling of a microbe possible. This type of test has a high degree of sensitivity and provides rapid and specific results.

FACT

With its ability to isolate small fragments associated with any microbe, PCR testing has moved to the forefront of candida testing. PCR testing can also be used with blood and urine samples, but that is not commonly done with candida testing.

Instructions in the kit may ask you to limit certain foods and medications, including antibiotics, probiotics, antacids, antifungals, brewer's yeasts, suppositories, enemas, and laxatives.

Blood Tests

Many doctors commonly order a blood workup to test for candida. These tests are readily available at many labs and easily ordered. If you have an aversion to needles or difficulty getting to a lab, this may not be your best option. Blood tests generally have a faster turn-around time than stool or urine testing.

These tests will try to identify the body's response to the presence of candida in the blood via production of substances known as antibodies or immunoglobulins. Antibodies are produced by the white blood cells in response to infections and other foreign substances that the body doesn't recognize. The three main antibodies associated with candida blood testing are IgA, IgG, and IgM. IgA is associated with immune responses that involve mucous cells, which are highly present in the digestive tract, lungs, sinuses, and vaginal surfaces. IgG, the smallest antibody, is also the most common antibody present throughout the body's fluids. In general, IgG antibodies indicate an infection that has been around for a while. IgM, the largest antibody present, is typically associated with recent infections.

Based on the antibody found in the blood tests, the lab will be able to determine if the candida infection is more recent, long-standing, or involves the mucous tissues. It is possible to have any combination of the three antibodies. For example, an old candida infection that is currently very active could cause both IgG and IgM to show up. IgA and mucous involvement could be present as well. An additional antibody, known as IgE, measures allergic responses and is used by some doctors when checking for candida, although much less frequently.

ESSENTIAL

Candida thrives on sugars and simple carbohydrates. When getting tested for candida, having eaten a meal high in simple carbohydrates (such as pastas, breads, and sugars) may help reveal an infection that would be less obvious if you were following a candida diet.

Antibodies are assisted in fighting infections by proteins that make up the body's complement system. They complement, or assist, the body in fighting infections by binding to the cells of candida and other microbes. Complement proteins will poke holes in the candida's cell wall, causing it to swell, rupture, and collapse. The presence of this complement complex combined with candida can be measured by another blood test called the Candida Immune Complex. This test will usually measure the Ig antibody levels as well. Some doctors consider this test to be more reliable than the antibody test. A combination of both tests is probably better than either one alone. Antibody testing is not limited to blood testing and can be done with saliva, urine, and stool tests as well.

Urine Tests

Urine testing tries to isolate candida in the urine, the presence of candida antibodies, or the metabolic markers of candida's presence in the body. The Great Plains Laboratories use the Organic Acid test to check urine for by-products of candida's metabolism or chemical processes. One candida by-product, a sugar called arabinose, is a reliable measure of candida activity. Director of Great Plains Laboratories Dr. William Shaw maintains that "a large percentage of chronically ill and autistic patients have candida metabolites in the urine that contribute significantly to symptoms, which can vary from person to person. . . ." In Shaw's opinion, the metabolic pathways that he has identified as abnormal may contribute to the symptoms of autistic spectrum disorders, fibromyalgia, chronic fatigue, and other neuro-degenerative disorders. His findings indicate that oxalic acid can precipitate in the tissues causing vulvodynia (chronic vaginal pain), where candida has infected the tissues of the labia, vagina, and urethra. According to Shaw, "oxalic acid can precipitate in any tissue (not just in the urogenital tract and kidneys) and potentially cause unexplained pain such as described by fibro-myalgia patients."

Like the stool test, the urine test doesn't require seeing a doctor and can be done at home. A collection kit will be sent to your home with instructions to limit fluid intake after 6:00 the evening before providing the sample to avoid diluted urine. The urine should be yellow in appearance. Women are asked to avoid collecting during their menstrual cycle. You can then mail the sample back to the lab in the packaging provided.

QUESTION

Are there candida tests for children?
Children can use the same tests as adults. Most of the same collection requirements apply and test results will be similar to those of adults. In the case of collecting a urine sample, a pediatric-size bag can be used. Overprescription of antibiotics is a common problem with children and creates a foundation for fungal candida.

Saliva Tests

Saliva testing may very well be the easiest test in terms of collection. Two methods are usually offered. The kit includes a cotton roll, which is placed in the mouth until it is saturated. Then the cotton roll is returned to the vial and sealed. Another method is to collect the saliva directly into the vial and then seal it. All samples should be refrigerated and mailed within three days of collection in the envelopes provided. If you have difficulty producing saliva, rinse your mouth with cold water a few minutes before collecting the sample.

Samples are usually collected between meals to avoid contamination with food particles. On the day of collection, avoid onions, garlic, caffeine, and cruciferous vegetables like cauliflower, cabbage, and broccoli. An hour before collection, avoid eating, brushing the teeth, using mouthwash, and smoking. Saliva tests may evaluate the presence of the antibodies: IgA, IgG, and IgM. They can also show inflammatory markers and test for the presence of the candida by-product, D-arabitol. Saliva testing is not as common as stool, blood, and urine testing, but it can be an excellent way to cross-reference candida's presence and effects.

Combined Testing

The best diagnostic evaluation is achieved by using several tests. Each of the methods mentioned earlier is most specific for the tissues from which the samples are collected. Having the results of two or three tests can present a more accurate picture of candida's presence. When combined with signs and symptoms, a history of antibiotic use, and any results from following a candida diet, these results will provide a wealth of information. No one test is able to reliably indicate candida's presence or absence, so for those people who wish to be accurate before proceeding with a plan, a combination of the tests is best advised.

The Spit Test

The name of this test, the Spit Test, is a dead giveaway as to its legitimacy. It was originally popularized as a marketing tool to convince as many people as possible that they had candida. The ease and instant ability to determine the presence of candida was a strong selling point. No labs, no costs, and no doctor visits were required. The instructions for administering the test were to "spit" into a glass of water first thing in the morning. If the saliva/mucus began to descend into the water and form threads, or what they called "legs," it was a positive indicator of candida. The threads, or legs, are created by increased mucous secretions, which are thicker than normal saliva due to the body's response to a foreign substance, candida. The problem with this diagnostic approach is that increased mucous secretions can just as easily be due to the following substances:

- Airborne allergies
- Bacteria
- Barometric pressure changes
- Chemicals
- Cold weather
- Dehydration
- Emotions
- Food allergies
- Heavy metals
- Molds
- Parasites
- Stress
- Viruses
- Yeast

The likelihood that several of these factors are present to some degree is extremely high. Most people are very dehydrated first thing in the morning due to seven to eight hours without fluid consumption. Bacteria, mold, virus, yeasts, fungi, chemicals, and heavy metals are all present in the body. The major detoxification organs are very active while the body rests and repairs itself, which can lead to increased mucous secretions as a protective response as toxins are released from the tissues and escorted out of the body.

ALERT

While the Spit Test may be harmless enough, if you have candida and determine via the test that you don't have it, you could end up wasting time and money investigating unrelated causes. Assessing everything together and getting the opinion of a health-care provider, if necessary, seems the better course of action.

Trusting the Tests

The complexity of the body's intestinal flora, immune system, physiology, anatomy, and the integration that exists among all of these factors makes testing a hit-and-miss proposition. In addition, testing has certain drawbacks that should be considered before investing time and finances.

Specificity

Candida tests are not specific enough. The current tests check only for the presence of the organism. They don't distinguish between the yeast and fungal forms. Since the fungal form creates the problems associated with candida, a positive test result should only indicate that this form was found. Unfortunately, a positive test could indicate that only the normal yeast form was present. The PCR testing format attempts to measure the number of candida present in the test sample. A high number can be a better indicator of candida overgrowth, and thus a fungal infection.

FACT

The PCR (polymerase chain reaction) test represented a revolutionary advancement in scientific testing with its invention in 1983. It was initially a slow, labor-intensive process until the development of specific enzymes and automated machine processes. Today, the test is known for its fast turn-around time, ease of use, and reliability. PCR testing has played a vital role in the advancement of genetic and AIDS research.

Localization

Positive test results are positive only for the tissue being tested. A positive stool test indicates the presence of candida only in the large intestine. A negative stool test does not discount the presence of candida in other tissues. An infection that is localized to the brain tissues may not show up in the stool. This is also true for the blood, urine, and saliva tests and for direct cultures, as well.

Sensitivity

Each test has a degree of sensitivity that translates, to a degree, to reliability. Blood tests are generally considered to be the least sensitive test. Candida doesn't spend much time in the blood due to the larger presence of white blood cells in the circulatory system. Candida's goal is to get to the tissues, not spend its time traveling. The more time it spends on the circulatory highway, the more likely it is that the white blood cells will destroy it.

Low sensitivity translates to false negatives. A negative finding doesn't mean that candida isn't there; it can mean that the test didn't find it. High-sensitivity tests like the PCR stool tests may result in false positives. The test may only be detecting the normal yeast form. This is a good reason to have multiple tests. It's not unusual to have a negative stool test and a positive blood test. Even when direct cultures of tissues have been negative, a blood test was positive. Each testing format has its Achilles' heel.

Cost

Candida testing can be costly. If you have a test done before following any candida program, then have the same test done upon completion to determine your success with the program. PCR stool tests tend to cost just under $500. Doing that twice gets to be pricey.

Investing finances in the treatment of candida may be a better way to spend your money. Some people choose less-expensive blood tests. Others use the testing for confirmation prior to following any candida plan and then gauge the success of the program by changes in their symptoms, conditions, and overall levels of health. This approach appears to be a good compromise that produces successful results. Whichever route you choose, testing offers a viable option but has certain limitations. Being aware of the limitations can help you avoid misunderstanding the test results.

As technology advances, better testing options will become available. Until then, current tests will have to do. Even with their imperfections, they represent significant advancements over past technologies and can be a great tool in diagnosing candida.

CHAPTER 4

Treating Candida

There are a variety of treatment options to address candida. Although treatment doesn't typically require a doctor's supervision, unless medications are involved, some people are more comfortable having the help of a qualified physician. If your condition is more complicated, getting professional advice can be a great place to start. However, there are plenty of other options that don't necessarily require supervision and can safely be done at home. Typically, the most successful treatments are the natural ones.

Medications

It's typical to think of medications as the best option for treating health challenges in today's world. The history of antifungal drugs is relatively short, as they were developed as a result of advances in modern medicine. Most doctors are familiar with a few of these drugs and will recommend them based on their experiences. A doctor will weigh the risks and benefits of using each medication. Based on your case history and test results, she will decide which medication is best for you and prescribe the dose she determines is sufficient. Should your problem continue, you will need to see her for a follow-up visit to determine if you need more of the same medication or a different one.

ALERT

Communicate any problems that you're having with medications directly to your doctor. Pay attention to how your body responds and don't hesitate to let him know. Other pre-existing conditions and diseases may not allow the use of certain drugs.

Be prepared for your visit. Write down all your medications, supplements, and personal health events in advance.

Amphotericin B

One of the oldest antifungal medications available, amphotericin B was first developed in the 1950s. Some doctors may still prefer to use this medication based on their experience with it. As with all antifungal drugs, the longer they have been around, the more unlikely they are to be effective, for the simple reason that fungi adapt quickly. Amphotericin targets the fat found in candida's cell wall, causing the inner components of the cell to leak out. Although this drug is still a standard choice in treating candida, it has significant associated toxicity.

Azoles

First developed in 1944, this class of drugs has several versions. The azoles tend to be one of the better-known class of antifungals, with recognizable brands like Diflucan, Nizoral, and Sporanox. Azoles try to block candida's ability to produce those fats necessary for the cell wall membrane. Some studies have shown that azoles are better tolerated and more effective than amphotericin B. Both classes of drugs have significant toxicity associated with their use, but azoles have less.

QUESTION

What are some of the side effects of these drugs?
Azole drugs are known to cause liver damage at varying dosages. Lab tests are the best way to determine liver problems, but if you are experiencing swelling anywhere in the body, tightness in the chest, a yellowish tinge in the whites of your eyes, stomach pain, skin rashes, fevers, chills, or loss of appetite, consult your doctor. Be aware of any changes as there are many other side effects associated with these drugs.

Due to the similarities between fungal cells and human cells, there is some concern that they can affect the body's ability to produce the cholesterol needed for human cell walls to function properly. If you take azole drugs for any time, it is important to have periodic evaluations of your liver function.

Nystatin

Nystatin is commonly used for many candida infections. Like amphotericin B, nystatin binds to the fat in candida's cell walls, causing them to leak. It has a safer record of use than other antifungal drugs. While other antifungals work systemically, nystatin is effective primarily in the intestinal tract. This excludes it as a choice in systemic fungal infections, although it may still have a lesser effect. Nystatin is commonly used prophylactically in patients with AIDS, or cancer, or needing organ transplants. It is a common choice in cases of oral and vaginal candida infections.

Some applications can also be used topically. Most doctors prescribe nystatin to outpatients due to its low toxicity profile. Side effects are usually limited to nausea, diarrhea, and vomiting. Anything else should be reported to your doctor at once.

Echinocandins

Echinocandins are designed to interfere with the production of sugars needed for candida's cell wall membranes. Developed in 2002, this is one of the newer classes of antifungals on the market. The echinocandins are designed for intravenous injection, which limits their practical use for most people. Like all antifungals, their initial response was good, but rapidly developing resistance has already begun and the usefulness of this class of drugs will eventually be outdated. Some common side effects include facial swelling, rashes, tightness in the chest, and liver toxicity in certain cases.

A 2012 study at Stanford University found that the average number of side effects for medications today is more than 300 per medication. Prior to this finding, it was believed that the average number of side effects per medication was only 68.

Due to the rapidly evolving development of antifungal resistance with all antifungal drugs, the search for new solutions is ongoing. Newer antifungals are being designed with less toxicity, but side effects still remain part of their use. Side effects from antifungals commonly include suppression of the immune system, which can lead to a worsening of the individual's condition. Each time a candida cell is destroyed, it releases its components into the surrounding tissues, which leads to a strong inflammatory response that can increase the severity of some symptoms and conditions. Unlike other natural choices, the use of medications always has associated risks.

If you choose to use medications to treat fungal candida, don't forget to follow a candida diet.

Herbs

The use of herbs has arguably the longest history in the treatment of candida. Some sources cite references from 3500 B.C. While medications will almost always be the treatment of choice in life-threatening situations, herbs are more likely to be the choice for people affected with candida.

In nature, fungus breaks down dead plant matter, therefore all plants have an antifungal pharmacy that prevents this from happening while they are still alive. As a result, the variety of plants and herbs available in treatment as antifungals is enormous. Plants vary from continent to continent, as the composition of the soils and available nutrients change. Oregano, a commonly used antifungal herb, can have different potencies and effects when grown in the Mediterranean as compared to when grown in Asia or the United States. Minor changes from one ecosystem to another can produce more or less potent forms of this herb.

Nature adapts to the demands placed on it in each location. Fortunately, with the technological advances in travel, agriculture, and the Internet, many herbs are readily available in the United States or Europe. The use of herbs and plants was originally part of the curriculum in medical schools. Even though medications are now synthetically produced, still more than 6,000 compounds used to make medicines are derived from Mother Nature.

Garlic

Garlic is perhaps the most popular herb for a variety of conditions. Apart from its use for keeping colds, the flu, and cancer at bay, garlic is a potent antifungal and antibacterial. Its first use was recorded more than 7,000 years ago. Garlic is one of the best examples of Hippocrates' dictum: "Let food be thy medicine and medicine be thy food." Hippocrates also first prescribed garlic for healing a variety of conditions.

So far, it appears that allicin, the active compound found in garlic, is responsible for its antifungal effects. Allicin, combined with antifungal drugs, has been shown to be more effective than the drugs used alone. One possible drawback is the compound's short-lived activity in the body, necessitating its ongoing usage to be maximally effective.

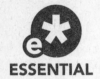

Garlic is sold as a supplement in capsule form. Dosages vary from 50 mg to 600 mg per capsule. One common recommended dosage is one 600-mg capsule, three times a day.

Oregano

The use of oregano dates back to the ancient Greeks, but it didn't find its way to the United States until World War II. Oregano is commonly used to flavor foods, especially Italian cuisine. The herb's active antifungal ingredients include thymol, terpenes, acetates, and carvacrol. Oregano also demonstrates antibacterial and antiviral properties. As a supplement, it commonly comes in an oil-based form, although the dried form is also available. Oil forms are available as a liquid or as a gel cap. Recommended dosages vary, but starting low and working your way up is a good rule of thumb. As a liquid, oregano is taken at one to three drops in 1 teaspoon of virgin coconut oil, extra-virgin olive oil, or almost any cold-pressed oil. In a gel cap, start with one capsule, one to two times a day. There's never a need to rush; proceed slowly and see how your body responds.

Grapefruit Seed Extract

Discovered in the 1970s, grapefruit seed extract has shown good results in studies, although there is some controversy around whether the pure extract is effective against fungal candida. Studies have shown that grapefruit seed extract is commonly contaminated with chemicals that are more likely to provide its antifungal effects.

Although commonly thought of as a natural extract, grapefruit seed extract requires enough processing that it probably qualifies as more of a synthetic. The entire product is effective against fungus, but the pure extract is not.

Pau d'Arco

Over the centuries, pau d'arco, also known as lapacho, has had a long history of use among descendants of the Inca and indigenous tribes of the Amazon rainforest. This herb is considered beneficial for a multitude of conditions that include candida, cancer, diabetes, parasites, viruses, allergies, and arthritis. Pau d'arco is a strong stimulator of the immune system.

Used in candida treatments, it can strongly inhibit candida, balance the blood sugar, reduce inflammation, and boost the immune system. Pau d'arco is generally supplied as a supplement or extract. If you would rather boil your herbs, you can also order the bark. As a supplement, each capsule will contain approximately 1,000 mg; the dosage is two capsules, one to three times a day. As an extract, you'll take 2 ml, one to three times a day. It also comes as a tea that you can sip throughout the day. Start slowly and work your way up.

Olive Leaf Extract

Olive leaves come from the same plant that provides olive oil. Its use dates back thousands of years to the Greeks and Romans. Like pau d'arco, olive leaf extract has been recommended for candida, inflammation, diabetes, viral and bacterial infections, healthy hearts, and high blood pressure. In ancient times, it was considered to be a cure for everything. This may have had more to do with early marketing techniques than actual cures, but its history of healing many conditions is impressive, nonetheless.

Olive leaf extract is an excellent all-around addition to anyone's daily diet. Its antioxidant potential is higher than that of green teas. It has a strong impact on viruses, making it an effective choice to fight colds and flu.

ESSENTIAL

Herbs are designed to inhibit fungus, not destroy it. Some people mistakenly believe that herbs must be rotated to avoid the resistance that develops with medications. Resistance is caused when a medication tries to kill an organism. Herbs don't produce that effect. As a result, they can be used on an ongoing basis.

Olive leaf extract is commonly available as a supplement or a liquid extract. As a supplement, it comes in 250-mg to 500-mg capsules. Recommended dosages are 500 mg to 1,000 mg per day. The dosage is the same for the liquid extract form. Some extracts can contain as much as 5,000 mg per serving, so go slowly and work your way up.

Black Walnut

Traditionally, this herb is more commonly associated with the elimination and control of parasites, but it has demonstrated moderate activity against fungal candida. Researchers at the University of Mississippi in 1990 showed that black walnut was as effective as some common antifungal medications. It has a long history of use against candida as well.

Black walnut is available as a supplement and in a tincture form, which is derived from the green hulls. The recommended dosage for the supplement is one capsule twice a day. Gradually increase the dosage over time. In the tincture form, recommended dosages can start as low as one drop per day, increasing over time to two teaspoons daily. Too much too soon can produce a laxative effect.

Tea Tree Oil

Tea tree oil, also known as melaleuca oil, has been around for thousands of years. It has great antiseptic qualities and many people tout its antifungal effects. This oil saw increased popularity during World War II, when it was given to soldiers to treat infections. It fell out of popular use with the beginning of the antibiotic era but eventually enjoyed a resurgence in popularity. Studies have shown that melaleuca has a moderate ability in preventing candida's conversion. As yet, it hasn't been shown to have a systemic effect on candida and is currently used mostly as a topical antifungal for skin and nail infections.

QUESTION

Is one herb better than another for treating candida?
The effects can vary from person to person and may depend on the quality of the herbs and other factors. Fortunately, several companies produce products that contain a combination of these herbs, so you don't have to rely on the effects of just one plant.

Tea tree oil is commonly available in a liquid form and also in capsule forms that combine several antifungal herbs. Recommended dosages for the liquid form are one to two drops applied topically. There is still some debate on its effectiveness internally as an antifungal.

Rosemary

Rosemary has shown a protective effect against changes to DNA. This is significant given the toxic world that exists today and the presence of many chemicals that are known to cause mutations. Rosemary has shown effectiveness against even drug-resistant strains of candida. Aside from using it to treat candida and protecting your genes, you may also find it useful for bacterial infections, memory, skin rashes, arthritis, nerve and muscle pain, poor circulation, high blood pressure, and the dreaded halitosis (bad breath). Rosemary is available as a liquid and in combination formulas of herbal supplements in its leaf form. The recommended dosages vary enough that it is best to follow the literature accompanying each product.

Cinnamon

Cinnamon has shown significant effectiveness against candida in research studies. It has also demonstrated effectiveness in the treatment of diabetes, Alzheimer's disease, poor circulation, and colon cancer. Certain components have also been shown to have antiviral effects. Adding cinnamon to foods can slow down the speed at which the stomach releases food and thus help reduce a rapid rise in blood sugars.

Anyone taking blood sugar or blood-thinning medications may need to take smaller amounts of cinnamon due to its ability to enhance the benefits of both types of medication. Always consult your doctor. Even though herbs have been enjoyed safely for thousands of years, medications have only been around for a few decades.

Cinnamon is commonly available as a supplement in dosages of 500 mg to 1,000 mg per capsule. The recommended intake for treating candida is usually 500 mg per meal. Always monitor the effect of anything you're taking.

Thyme

Thyme was often given to soldiers before battle to encourage bravery. Some people are likely to view a candida diet as a personal battle against a lifetime of bad food choices, so this use may still be appropriate. Thyme has been used as an antiseptic, an aphrodisiac, and an embalming agent, with the latter giving rise to its use as a preservative for foods.

In healing, thyme has been used for sore throats, coughs, lung congestion, asthma, digestive imbalances, rheumatism, clearing the liver, boosting the immune system, purifying water, and, of course, candida. Like all herbs, thyme has multiple components that have been shown to affect many conditions. It is available as the dried leaf in capsules and as a liquid. The recommended dosage in capsule form is two capsules, one to three times a day. As a liquid, fifteen to thirty drops in water, three times a day. Some people mix the thyme in water and drink it as a tea. Start slowly and work your way up to higher dosages.

Cloves

Cloves, appropriately enough, are said to originate from the Spice Islands. Their use is found in Chinese and Ayurvedic medicine texts dating back centuries. As they did with other spices, empires sought to control the trade of cloves. This spice has demonstrated antibacterial, antifungal, antiviral, and antiparasitic activity. Cloves are more commonly used for their antiparasitic effects. Dentists have used cloves to reduce tooth pain. Other healing uses include digestive imbalances, vomiting, diarrhea, headaches, nail fungus, athlete's foot, and depression. Research studies have proved the effectiveness of cloves against candida. Some studies cite greater effectiveness than antifungal drugs.

Cloves are available as a supplement in capsule and liquid versions. One 450-mg capsule, one to three times a day, is recommended. In the liquid form, the dosage is fifteen to twenty drops in water, one to three times a day.

Fennel

Every part of the fennel plant—seeds, stems, flowers, oil, and bulb—has been put to use since the time of Pliny in ancient Rome. Fennel has been recommended for asthma, congestion, breast enlargement, digestive imbalances, libido enhancement, colic, and the occasional snakebite. Organs that benefit from fennel include the lungs, kidneys, liver, small and large intestine, and spleen. As an antifungal, the essential oil of fennel, like the essential oils of many plants, has demonstrated high antifungal activity against candida. As a supplement, fennel is commonly available as an essential oil. The seeds and other edible parts provide some antifungal activity, as well as other benefits. For example, taking 2–3 g of the seeds one to three times a day has been shown to alleviate digestive imbalances. Fennel is commonly found in colic formulas. It is also available as a tea.

ESSENTIAL

Essential oils typically contain potent extracts of the plants they are derived from. As a result, the dosages are much less than for the plant itself. To avoid side effects, be sure to follow carefully the instructions that are provided with all essential oils.

The list of herbs used as antifungals is more extensive than what is provided here and can vary from country to country. It includes lemongrass, anise, peppermint, spearmint, and mint. Enter the name of the herb you are interested in, followed by the word *antifungal* on an Internet search, and you will most likely find a scientific reference for its use against candida and other fungi. There are a wide variety of choices available. As discussed earlier, the effect of plants in nature is to inhibit fungus, so while herbs make an excellent and safe addition to any candida program, their best usage is in conjunction with other antifungal choices. Many studies are already testifying to the ability of herbs to make the use of antifungal medications more effective. Antifungal medication dosages can be reduced as well if they are taken in conjunction with herbs.

Probiotics

The word *probiotic* means "for life." These micro-organisms have been in use as long as fermented foods have been on the planet. Probiotics were formally recognized by Russian scientist Élie Metchnikoff in 1907, and the identification of different probiotics and the exploration of their benefits have continued ever since.

Despite scientific advances, the medical world is only beginning to identify the vast majority of microbes that inhabit the human body. The small amount that they do know about a limited number of these microbes has led to the creation and marketing of several products and foods formulated with bacteria and yeast. Unfortunately, since most of the bacteria in the body are unable to survive outside of it, they cannot be used in probiotic formulas. Nonetheless, key insights into the beneficial function of various probiotic species and strains have resulted from the research. Probiotics, for example, have an indirect antifungal effect.

FACT

The best method to ensure that a patient receives the highest number of probiotic species appears to be a fecal transplant. In this treatment, a fecal sample is taken from a healthy donor and implanted into a recipient. Its success rate against antibiotic-induced, life-threatening diarrhea is approximately 96 percent.

As with herbs, probiotics have demonstrated a higher degree of safety than medications. The mixture of species and strains vary from formulation to formulation. The following discussion examines the key types of probiotics and their role in establishing a healthy ecosystem inside the body, which will be the main deterrent against the overgrowth of candida.

Lactobacillus

The *Lactobacillus* genus of bacteria is one of the main probiotics to inhibit the growth of candida. These micro-organisms form lactic acid from sugars, such as the lactose sugar commonly found in milk products. Lactose intolerance usually means that an individual is deficient in these friendly bacteria. The lactic acids produced by *Lactobacillus* are a major inhibitor of the growth of fungal candida. Scientific research has found additional benefits including the reduction of skin disorders, allergies, high cholesterol, and diarrhea, and boosting weak immune systems. Studies have also shown that consumption of *Lactobacillus* probiotics has lessened the incidence of cancer. Most fermented foods owe a lot of their health benefits to the *Lactobacillus* species that they contain.

QUESTION

May I eat fermented foods on a candida diet?
Fermented foods provide higher amounts of probiotics than most probiotic formulas. Although this would appear to be a great reason for including them on the diet, fermented foods also contain high amounts of histamine, which can initially exacerbate many conditions. Adding them in on week 9 of the diet plan is often best.

Lactobacillus probiotics come formulated as powders, capsules, tablets, and solutions. An upper limit on the number or amount of probiotics an individual consumes daily has not been established. Some people are concerned that certain species or strains may not pass the acid levels of the stomach and should only be consumed in a capsule form. This has not been shown to be an issue.

Bifidobacterium

The *Bifidobacterium* genus of bacteria takes up residence in the large intestine, while the *Lactobacillus* genus is more commonly associated with the stomach, small intestine, oral cavity, and vaginal tissues. Like the *Lactobacillus*, the *Bifidobacterium* also ferment sugars to produce lactic acid. So far, it appears that these bacteria are also able to break down other plant fibers. They are believed to be one of the primary forms of bacteria found in breastmilk and play an important role in the development of a healthy child. *Bifidobacterium* produce short-chain fatty acids that exert additional antifungal effects and help nourish and protect the cells of the wall of the intestinal tract. Additional effects include immune-boosting potential and the ability to reduce inflammation in the body's tissues. These bacteria come formulated as powders, capsules, tablets, and solutions. There is no set upper limit on the daily amount to consume. If taking too much at first produces gas and bloating, reduce the initial dosage for a few days and then try increasing it once more.

Streptococcus thermophilus

This particular species of probiotic is found readily in yogurts and in almost all probiotic formulas. Like *Lactobacillus* and *Bifidobacterium*, it produces lactic acid from sugars. It has been used in fermented foods for thousands of years, especially in yogurts and cheeses. This lactic-acid bacterium has been shown to help weight gain and growth in children and to control antibiotic-induced diarrhea. Additionally, it helps reduce inflammation in the intestinal tract and protect against antibiotic-resistant bacteria like *E. coli*.

ALERT

The use of probiotics has had an excellent safety record for centuries. Some concern exists around the use of probiotics in individuals with severe immune-system suppression, such as occurs with HIV, cancer, and when taking immunosuppressive drugs. Risks in this area are unclear and should be evaluated by a physician on a case-by-case basis.

Streptococcus thermophilus is found in fermented foods and is sold as a part of powders, capsules, tablets, and solutions.

Multistrain Probiotics

A key to the overall health of the digestive tract lies in the diversity of organisms present. Although individual probiotic strains have noted benefits, it is the effect of all of the bacteria together that will have the greatest impact.

A multistrain probiotic formula offers the best solution to controlling candida and improving health. Good formulas will contain a wide variety of strains to enhance the overall effect and benefits. Formulas with ten or more strains per capsule are stronger and more beneficial. There is no upper limit to the amount of probiotics that can be consumed daily, but you should always work within your body's comfort levels. Probiotics are living organisms, and all formulas will contain a food source as well. Inulin is a long-chain sugar that is the optimum food for probiotics. A short-chain version, called FOS (fructo-ologosaccharides), may cause allergic reactions and is more likely to feed both the good and the bad bacteria. A probiotic with inulin is a better choice.

Fatty Acids

Fatty acids are the individual building blocks that make up the oils used for cooking. Olive oil, for instance, is composed of oleic, linoleic, palmitic, stearic, and linolenic fatty acids. With a long history of use, fatty acids provide the best of all worlds when it comes to candida treatments. Derived from plants, fatty acids provide many of the same benefits. Many fatty acids are as effective as medications without the side effects or other risks.

ESSENTIAL

Fatty acids have a more concentrated antifungal effect than the oils in which they are found. Follow recommended dosages for each fatty acid.

The human body produces its own armory of fatty acids, and many are similar to those produced in plants. Three fatty acids—caprylic acid, undecenoic acid, and lauric acid—have been found to be very useful in the treatment of candida. They will produce the best results and can even be combined with any of the other methods mentioned here. The following sections will discuss their potency and effectiveness.

Caprylic Acid

Caprylic acid is the most commonly available form of fatty acids in the treatment of candida. It is derived from coconut oil. Any antifungal effect of coconut oil is usually attributed to its caprylic acid content, although the oil also contains lauric acid; each fatty acid present will likely have some degree of added antifungal activity. Long-term use of this fatty acid may produce some problems for the kidneys. Short-term use of four to six weeks is considered acceptable. Otherwise, caprylic acid is usually considered a safe choice. It has been found in human breastmilk in very small quantities.

It commonly comes in dosages of 500 mg to 1,000 mg. The recommended daily dose varies from about 1,000 mg to 3,000 mg a day.

Undecenoic Acid

Undecenoic acid is the reigning king of candida treatments. Distilled from the oil of castor beans, it can also be found as a component of human sweat along with other fatty acids.

Its long history of use against fungal candida dates to just after the introduction of antibiotics. Early experiments found undecenoic acid to be useful against a wide variety of conditions associated with candida. Skin disorders were among the first links to fungal-induced imbalances created by the use of antibiotics in 1949. Early doses of undecenoic acid were very high but produced dramatic results. Modern dosages are much smaller due to the addition of a dietary protocol that reduces the food sources that candida readily feeds upon.

Undecenoic acid was found to be more effective than lauric acid, and as much as six times more effective than caprylic acid. Later studies showed that combining undecenoic acid with calcium, zinc, or magnesium produced a salt form that was more than thirty times as effective as caprylic acid. Unfortunately, the salt form is more dependent on the pH present in the tissues. Its greatest effect is limited to acidic environments and is not capable of addressing fungal candida issues throughout the body. Many people have found undecenoic acid useful for ringworm and other types of fungal-oriented skin conditions. It has also demonstrated some effectiveness against the herpes simplex virus but is better known for its antifungal properties.

Undecenoic acid is typically combined with extra-virgin olive oil in a gel cap at doses of 50 mg per gel cap. The typical dosage recommendation is 250 mg, or five gel caps, three times a day, for a total of 750 mg daily. The typical length of treatment with undecenoic acid in this form is eight weeks.

Continued use has not been shown to create problems, and some people take a maintenance dosage of 250 mg a day.

Lauric Acid

Lauric is the least popular and probably the last choice in fatty acids for treating fungal candida. Although studies have shown it to be more effective than caprylic acid, its popularity hasn't advanced. Like caprylic acid, it is found in coconut oil and breastmilk, as well as in plants. Lauric acid is noted more for its antiviral effects than its antifungal effects. A common ester of lauric acid, known as monolaurin, is sold for its antiviral and immune-boosting properties.

Lauric acid is commonly available in the monolaurin form in dosages of 500 mg to 600 mg. The recommended daily dosage as an antifungal is approximately 2,000 mg per day.

Fatty acids can produce the best results when treating fungal candida. They are safe and effective as a stand-alone choice but can also be combined with herbs, medications, probiotics, and other available choices. Always let your doctor know when you are combining anything with medications. Your doctor may not be familiar with your antifungal choices, but informing her that you are doing something else can then allow her to do more research into your choices.

What Not to Use to Treat Candida

The treatments listed in these next few sections may seem to be workable choices that can produce good results when fighting candida, but their long-term impact may be negative.

Colloidal Silver

Colloidal silver is a form of silver that has been broken up into very small particles and suspended in a solution. Silver has a long history of use against infections. Colloidal silver is known primarily for its antibacterial effects. Some studies have shown effectiveness against the microbial films that can surround and protect candida. These biofilms are composed mostly of bacterial cells.

Colloidal silver has not been shown to be safe for all of the bacteria that line the body. It may destroy beneficial bacteria that play an important role as well. Affecting the composition of the body's bacterial flora may have detrimental effects that won't become apparent for years. While colloidal silver may be a superior choice to antibiotics, it doesn't appear to be as safe as the fatty acids.

Turpentine

Most people immediately think that turpentine is a dangerous substance to ingest for any reason. However, there are different types of turpentine available. The version that most people think about is a poison and may cause vomiting. There is another version, distilled from tree resin, that has a long history of use. Traditionally, it has been used as an antiparasitic, as well as for lung congestion and snakebite. Turpentine was a handy home remedy that has been credited with saving lives.

ALERT

Ingesting even small amounts of turpentine can be fatal! This poison is commonly consumed by children.

Turpentine's effect as an antimicrobial against all types of infections is primarily anecdotal. Although it may be effective against candida and other bugs, its known toxicity is likely to create other imbalances that could be damaging to the body in some other way that may not be readily apparent.

Lufenuron

Lufenuron is a flea medication designed to disrupt the synthesis of chitin in the shells of insects. Since chitin makes up a moderate portion of candida's cell wall membrane as well, Lufenuron might seem like a good choice. That logic, however, does not take into consideration the ability of candida to adapt to such drugs.

Skin conditions attributed to candida and healed by taking Lufenuron are more likely due to its ability to affect certain enzymes rather than its effect on candida. One definitive study done at the University of California,

San Francisco, looked at the antifungal properties of Lufenuron and two other antifungal medications. The authors concluded, "Lufenuron does not appear to possess antifungal properties."

Chlorine

The antibacterial properties of chlorine are so well known that it is added to city water worldwide and used as a disinfectant in hospitals. Chlorine is a hazardous toxin and requires careful handling. As a healing agent, chlorine has been used in very dilute solutions (2 percent chlorine). Dioxychlor and MMS are dilute chlorine solutions that are promoted to treat infections.

Candida's resistance develops quickly. If these solutions are able to kill candida, the organism will adapt rapidly and their usefulness will be limited. Chlorine is a strong oxidizing agent; consumption has been linked to arterial disease.

Bacillus subtilis

This strain of bacteria has strong antifungal properties. It is not normally found in the human intestinal tract and does not appear to implant readily into the microflora. *B. subtilis* has also demonstrated an even stronger antibacterial effect. It has been used as the basis for the development of several antibiotics that are currently in use. Its antibiotic effect is likely to create more problems than it can solve.

CHAPTER 5

Blood-Related Issues Associated with Candida

Candida continues to be linked to more symptoms and conditions as technology enhances science's ability to reveal the hidden workings of this amazing organism. For example, inflamation is very often associated with candida and other conditions. As scientists discover more about inflammation's link to disease, they learn more about how candida can also be linked to these same conditions. Certain blood-related issues, for example, tend to show up more frequently with candida. Knowing what they are and how they can affect your health in many other ways can be helpful information.

Blood Sugar Imbalances

One common symptom of fungal candida's presence is the deregulation of blood sugar levels, also known as dysglycemia, which creates either high or low levels of blood sugar. Low levels of blood sugar are referred to as hypoglycemia, while high levels of blood sugar are referred to as hyperglycemia, or insulin resistance. With fungal candida, it is increasingly common to see both. Left untreated, the ever-increasing levels of high blood sugar can lead to diabetes, which is associated with obesity, strokes, blindness, heart attacks, circulation problems, and neurodegenerative diseases. Diabetes is a leading cause of mortality worldwide. Like a game of dominoes, candida plays a key role in setting in motion a series of events that leads to the body's inability to regulate blood sugar.

Blood Sugar

One of the main sources of fuel for all cells is glucose, which is generated by breaking down the carbohydrates found in foods. Carbohydrates can be simple or complex. Simple carbohydrates include breads, pastas, cereals, tortillas, crackers, and sweets. Complex carbohydrates include potatoes, yams, squash, and many vegetables. Simple carbohydrates tend to raise blood sugar, or glucose, levels faster than complex carbohydrates.

After absorption into the blood, glucose is then transported throughout the bloodstream to tissues and cells. The cells absorb the glucose with the help of insulin, a hormone that unlocks the door to the cells, allowing glucose to enter each one. When too much insulin is present, the level of glucose in the blood drops and the levels inside the cells increase. With too little insulin, or an inability of insulin to bind to the cells and "unlock the door," blood levels of glucose rise and cellular levels decrease. Both imbalances lead to sickness and disease. Knowing the signs of each one can help identify the presence of candida and determine how to address the imbalances.

Hypoglycemia

Low blood sugar is probably the most common problem associated with dysglycemia. As the potency of antibiotics and the number of incidences of candida infections have increased over the years, the incidence of hypoglycemia and hyperglycemia has also risen.

Signs of low blood sugar include feeling shaky, irritable, anxious, tired, moody, and craving sweets. Reactive hypoglycemia occurs when an individual goes too long without eating. The length of time can vary from person to person.

Standard blood tests don't adequately measure blood sugar imbalances, although they may hint at them. The gold standard for measuring these imbalances, and the most common way to assess for diabetes, is the Oral Glucose Tolerance Test (OGTT). A baseline, or initial test, is done to determine the person's current blood sugar levels. Then, the person is given a sugary solution to drink and his blood is drawn every thirty to sixty minutes over a three-hour period.

Side effects are minimal, but they may include nausea and lightheadedness, much like eating a large bag of Halloween candy. A sharp fall in blood sugar levels will be a positive indication of hypoglycemia. The sharper the drop, the more severe the hypoglycemia. Although there have been many criticisms of this test, a better laboratory test is not yet available. Many factors such as medications, stress, alcohol, smoking, inherited conditions, and health conditions involving the thyroid, liver, and pancreas may affect this test.

A functional assessment of hypoglycemia is based on whether the individual feels tired, moody, irritable, or anxious when going too long without food. If so, that's positive for reactive hypoglycemia. Most people who experience hypoglycemia will feel better just by eating, which helps to raise blood sugar levels temporarily. The inability to regulate the blood sugar can lead to those levels falling again. Once an individual enters an episode of reactive hypoglycemia, it can cause a chain reaction that affects hormones, the immune system, the adrenals, and the nervous system. Although eating will make the person feel better quickly, the chain reaction will continue unchecked for several hours. Symptoms associated with reactive hypoglycemia include:

- Hormonal imbalances that affect estrogen, testosterone, and thyroid hormones
- Immune-system dysregulation or suppression
- Adrenal symptoms such as fatigue, loss of libido, and an inability to handle stress
- Neurological issues such as anxiety, depression, headaches, and brain fog

A good candida program can help establish better regulation of blood sugar levels. A diet of whole foods can reverse blood sugar imbalances and diabetes. Since the imbalances associated with hypoglycemia can be severe enough to create dysfunction on a daily basis, it can be far better to address this through the Blood Sugar Protocol while following any candida plan.

The Blood Sugar Protocol requires eating a small handful of food every sixty minutes. Since fruit sugar can be hard to handle with blood sugar imbalances, it's best to eat a small amount of protein or vegetable. Celery is an excellent choice because it is easy to prepare, easy to carry, and doesn't go bad quickly.

QUESTION

May I follow the Blood Sugar Protocol while taking medications for diabetes?
The Blood Sugar Protocol should help create more stability with blood sugar levels and shouldn't interfere with the use of diabetic medications. By helping the body better regulate the highs and lows of blood sugar using the protocol, you may be able to reduce your medications. Check first with your doctor before changing the dosage of any of your medications.

A typical day might look like this: You get up at 7:00 A.M. and have a piece of celery right away. You get ready for your day and eat breakfast, all within an hour. An hour after breakfast, you have another piece of celery. An hour later, another piece. You continue this until bedtime. Since the body enters into a fasting state during sleep, it is not uncommon for people to wake up in the middle of the night when experiencing hypoglycemia. Waking up in a sweat can be another sign of hypoglycemia. Place a piece or two of celery on your nightstand, so that it is readily available should you wake up. Having a small piece of celery before going back to sleep can help the body meet its energy requirements and help you sleep better. Have a snack as soon as you get up for the day and follow the protocol. It is important to follow this protocol strictly for a period of four months. Doing so can eliminate a wide range of problems that interfere with a healthy, active lifestyle. When done in conjunction with any candida diet, the Blood Sugar Protocol can improve the speed at which positive changes take place in the body.

Hyperglycemia

Hyperglycemia is a state of high blood sugar. Most people aren't familiar with this term; it is frequently called prediabetes or insulin resistance. Prediabetes is marked by ever-increasing levels of blood sugar and is also known as intermediate hyperglycemia. Left untreated, it can lead to diabetes in only ten years. Using the standard blood test assessment, hyperglycemia is considered to be present when the blood levels of glucose range from 100–125. The normal blood sugar range is typically 70–100. Some consider the range for hyperglycemia to be too narrow.

ALERT

Never allow your doctor to prescribe medications based on the findings of one or two tests alone. Many factors can influence tests, including the stress of the doctor's visit and then the worry about the results. This is known as the "white coat" effect. One finding is an incident, two is a coincidence, and three or more is a trend. Prescriptions should be based on trends along with signs, symptoms, and other pertinent health history information.

Criticisms of the standard fasting blood-glucose testing and the Oral Glucose Tolerance Test led to the development of an additional test, the A1C, to help determine if prediabetes, or diabetes, is present. The A1C test measures the amount of glucose bound to hemoglobin in the red blood cells. Hemoglobin is the iron-bound protein that is responsible for transporting oxygen to cells and tissues throughout the body. Since red blood cells live for only thirty days, the A1C test helps provide an assessment of blood sugar levels over the ninety days before you take the test. The normal range is a reading below 5.7, hyperglycemia is 5.7 to 6.4, and diabetes is 6.5 and above. There are several criticisms of this test. It is possible to have a positive finding on the fasting glucose and a negative finding on the A1C, and vice versa. Remember that tests are only a snapshot in time; the results of several will tell a more accurate story.

Common symptoms associated with hyperglycemia include excessive thirst, frequent urination, fatigue, and headaches. The Blood Sugar Protocol can be used successfully with hyperglycemia and hypoglycemia. A good candida program can create incredible changes in blood sugar control.

Candida has a strong link to hyperglycemia. Researchers at the University of San Diego found that high levels of protease enzymes in the blood and tissues can cause prediabetes, high blood pressure, and immune-system suppression. Candida produces ten different protease enzymes, known as secreted aspartyl proteases (SAPs). Proteases break down protein-based structures in the body.

Insulin is a protein-based hormone and has attachments, or receptors, on its surface that bind to cells and allow blood sugar to enter the cell. These protease enzymes have been shown to cut off these receptors, leading to increased levels of blood sugar. As blood sugar levels increase or remain high, cell function suffers without sugar as a fuel source, leading to the symptoms of fatigue and headaches associated with hyperglycemia.

FACT

Prediabetes is rapidly closing in on 40 percent of the U.S. population. In 2002, it affected approximately 27 percent of thepopulation and increased to just over 34 percent in 2010, placing current estimates somewhere in the neighborhood of 37–38 percent. One article that appeared in the *Lancet Journal* projected that worldwide "more than 470 million people will have pre-diabetes by 2030."

Hyperglycemia and hypoglycemia are stepping stones to diabetes, but they can be reversed with the right approach and consistent effort. Modifying lifestyle through diet, detoxification, and exercise has been shown to improve and correct blood sugar imbalances.

Diabetes

Diabetes is a condition marked by high blood sugar levels due to decreased production of insulin by the pancreas, or an inability of the cells to use the insulin that is being produced. The World Health Organization predicts that diabetes will be the seventh-leading cause of death in the world by 2030. Currently, close to 3.5 million people die annually of complications related to diabetes. Symptoms include excessive thirst and urination, weight loss or gain, skin problems, candida infections, fatigue, blurred vision, and tingling or numbness in the hands and feet.

While hypoglycemia and hyperglycemia are imbalances that can lead to diabetes, diabetes is an imbalance that is increasingly associated with obesity, arthritis, psoriasis, cardiovascular diseases, Alzheimer's disease, and Parkinson's disease. These conditions have also been increasingly associated with candida due to the increased levels of inflammation that it produces.

Researchers from the University of California, Davis, and the University of Pennsylvania have linked psoriasis to diabetes. The mechanism involved appears to be inflammation and immune system dysregulation. The inflammation associated with psoriasis has been found to produce the insulin resistance seen in prediabetes and diabetes. Dr. Christina Zielinski, a researcher from the Institute for Research in Biomedicine, has found consistent links between candida, psoriasis, and the manufacture of inflammatory proteins, called cytokines, which are produced by white blood cells. These candida-stimulated cytokines have also been associated with arthritis, autoimmune disease, Crohn's disease, and cardiovascular and neurological diseases.

The incidence of candida infections is higher in diabetics. With blood sugar levels unregulated, diabetes becomes a feeding ground for candida and other pathogenic microbes. Researchers from the India Institute of Medical Sciences have shown that patients with diabetes are at an increased risk for oral and vaginal candida. Given that diabetes is a systemic problem that can suppress the immune system, diabetics are more vulnerable to infections that include candida and other pathogens. An abundant sugar supply and a suppressed immune system are two of the most powerful facilitators of fungal candida infections. If a diabetic takes an antibiotic and wipes out all the bacteria in the body within five to seven days, fungal candida within forty-eight hours is a foregone conclusion.

ESSENTIAL

Smoking is a bad habit for many reasons, and candida is another one of those reasons. Most smokers have candida problems. Diabetics who smoke are even more likely to have candida problems.

Science shows how candida is able to create diabetes and how diabetes, in turn, is able to support fungal candida overgrowth. Candida's ability to create problems in the body that help foster its continued growth and existence is uncanny. It reveals how advanced this organism is and how millions of years of evolution have equipped it to handle almost every environment it finds itself in.

Gestational Diabetes

Gestational diabetes is a temporary increase of blood sugar levels during the course of a pregnancy that usually resolves after delivery. Its presence during the pregnancy places the baby at risk. The cause is unknown at this time, but evidence points to an increase in insulin resistance by the cells. One possible cause could be candida. Researchers from Second Obstetrics and Gynecology Clinics, Ankara Education and Research Hospital in Turkey discovered that pregnant women with fungal candida have an impaired ability to handle glucose.

During pregnancy, a woman's immune system shifts toward an immune response that favors the birth of the baby and the growth of candida. The part of the immune system most responsible for eliminating fungal candida is the Th1 immune response. This response is suppressed during pregnancy;

it would try to end the pregnancy because the implanted egg is viewed as a foreign tissue.

Suppressing the immune response helps facilitate an ongoing pregnancy. Suppressing the Th1 immune response, however, causes an elevation in the Th2 immune response and candida's growth can become more pronounced. Pregnancy does not cause candida. It only reveals or exacerbates an infection that already exists by making it more symptomatic. Whether the Th1 or the Th2 immune response supports diabetes has yet to be determined. So far, it is known that candida supports diabetes and is frequently associated with pregnancies. At least for now, this appears to be a clearer link to gestational diabetes. Pregnant women with diabetes could benefit from better blood sugar regulation and may want to consider following the Blood Sugar Protocol. As a side note, an additional consideration regarding candida and pregnancy is infertility. Candida has been shown to be involved in several areas that can affect a woman's ability to get pregnant.

QUESTION

Can candida prevent pregnancies?
Many women who have done a candida plan have been able to conceive after a medical diagnosis of infertility. This has been achieved repeatedly in a clinical setting but has not yet been studied in a research setting.

Bacterial vaginosis, a condition marked by the presence of abnormal bacterial flora in the vaginal tissues, was shown to have a "significant association with infertility" by researchers in India (*www.ncbi.nlm.nih.gov*). Bacterial vaginosis can be related to fungal candida overgrowth, since candida can play a role in regulating which bacteria repopulate tissues after antibiotic use.

Candida has also been shown to inhibit the lactic acid–forming bacteria that are known to normally populate the vaginal tissues. Lactic acid–producing bacteria help prevent the growth of harmful bacteria associated with bacterial vaginosis. Additionally, a man's sperm causes an increased Th17 response by the woman's body. As Dr. Zielinski and other researchers have established, Th17 is also created by the presence of fungal candida.

The exact role of Th17 in infertility, miscarriages, and spontaneous abortions has not been clarified.

While the presence of sperm would be a temporary occurrence and not likely to cause infertility, a systemic fungal candida imbalance would increase inflammation on a more chronic basis and may play a role in infertility and miscarriages. As science continues to advance, medical doctors will have a better understanding of the role of candida in creating diabetes, and of diabetes' role in creating candida imbalances.

CHAPTER 6

Digestive Problems Associated with Candida

The long list of digestive problems commonly associated with fungal candida begins to sound like a television commercial after a while. If you have gas, bloating, indigestion, acid reflux, or an upset stomach, then you could have candida.

Low Levels of Hydrochloric Acid

Hydrochloric acid (HCl or stomach acid) is produced by cells within the stomach. Stomach acid is a mixture of hydrochloric acid, sodium chloride, potassium chloride, mucus, proteins, and enzymes. A complex series of reactions creates hydrochloric acid. The sight, smell, and ingestion of food, even the thought of food, causes an increased production of HCl, which helps neutralize pathogens, activate the enzyme pepsin for breaking down proteins, and assists with absorption of several other key nutrients. Low HCl levels are associated with a series of imbalances linked to many diseases, as well as to the loss of absorption of essential nutrients and cofactors. The common use of medicines not only exacerbates the effects of low HCl levels, it also creates and helps sustain more fungal candida overgrowth. As people age, their HCl levels decline, which predisposes them to conditions associated with low HCl levels and candida overgrowth.

Acid Reflux

Acid reflux has traditionally been treated as a condition caused by low levels of hydrochloric acid. These low levels lead to cycles of over- and underproduction of the acid. When an individual with normal levels eats, the resting levels of HCl increase mildly to handle the functions necessary for processing the food. When the meal is over, the hydrochloric acid returns to its normal resting level. When an individual has low HCl levels, a much larger increase in production is necessary to handle digestion. Once the food is processed, the low levels of HCl return. Overproduction of hydrochloric acid leads to acid reflux, or GERD (Gastro-Esophageal Reflux Disease).

FACT

The incidence of acid reflux, or heartburn, increases with age, escalating rapidly after age forty. Researchers from Beth Israel Hospital in Boston, Massachusetts, state that "20–40 percent of the adult population experience heartburn." The death rate is low, but the "quality of life can be significantly impaired."

A major factor in the overall function of the stomach, as elsewhere in the digestive tract, is the role of the bacterial flora. While the numbers of bacteria present in the stomach are lower than elsewhere in the intestinal tract, researchers from the University of Michigan Medical School have shown that these bacteria are "vital in promoting colonization resistance against *Candida albicans*." Once antibiotics have been taken, these bacteria are wiped out and fungal candida develops.

Fungal candida then helps reshape the composition of the stomach flora. This is especially true of the *Lactobacillus* bacteria, which is the most abundant species present in the stomach and helps produce acids that create a balanced, beneficial bacterial flora. The reshaping of the stomach flora has also been linked with the body's response to another normal bacterial resident of the stomach, *Helicobacter pylori* (*H. pylori*). Although associated with causing ulcers, gastritis, and stomach cancers, *H. pylori* also have a positive effect: a reduced incidence of asthma and allergies. How the body responds to *H. pylori* determines whether the bacteria's effect is beneficial or harmful. Altering the stomach flora with antibiotics determines which response takes place. Antibiotics and candida cause a significant shift in the stomach flora that can lead to acid reflux and other conditions related to low levels of hydrochloric acid. For decades, the standard treatment for acid reflux has been to take HCl pills or to use a weak acid, like apple cider vinegar, at mealtime to aid digestion.

Gastritis

Gastritis is another candida-related condition marked by inflammation of the stomach lining. Like acid reflux, it is marked by low levels of hydrochloric acid. *H. pylori* is also associated with gastritis, as low hydrochloric acid levels predispose the stomach to overgrowth and infection with these bacteria.

As few as seven days of antibiotic use has been shown to create gastritis. In a study appearing in *Infection and Immunity* (a peer-reviewed journal published by the American Society for Microbiology), researchers found that antibiotics alone were not enough to create gastritis. Having studied the effects of the antibiotic cefoperazone on the stomach flora, their findings state that "disturbance of the gastric bacterial community by cefoperazone alone was not sufficient to cause gastritis, *C. albicans* colonization was also needed." Given its basic association with gastritis, correcting imbalances of fungal candida holds promise as a logical way to address the condition.

Ulcers

An ulcer is often described as the erosion of the lining of the stomach, esophagus, or small intestine, but it can also apply to other tissues, such as the skin. Common symptoms may include upper abdominal pain that is worse between meals and at night or that is relieved by eating. These symptoms typically describe a peptic ulcer. The location will further differentiate the type of ulcer. In the stomach, it is a gastric ulcer; in the esophagus, an esophageal ulcer; and in the duodenum, a duodenal ulcer. *H. pylori* is linked to ulcers, and most treatments, unfortunately, involve antibiotics.

QUESTION

Are there any natural ways to treat high levels of hydrochloric acid?
Mixing ¼ teaspoon of baking soda in about 6 ounces of water, and drinking the mixture during episodes of heartburn or acid reflux can work as effectively as medications but without the associated side effects or damage. This is a quick fix. The best approach is to address the underlying causes of the condition.

Researchers from Jagiellonian University Medical College studied 158 patients with *H. pylori* infections and discovered fungal candida in 50 percent.

Nutrient Losses

Beginning in the 1970s, antacid medications were marketed directly to consumers. As a result, their popularity has increased. In recent years, Boxed Warnings (also known as Black Box Warnings) have started to appear on antacid medications warning of possible nutrient deficiencies. These warnings are used by the U.S. Food and Drug Administration (FDA) to alert consumers to serious adverse reactions or life-threatening risks associated with certain prescription drugs.

The first warning on antacids appeared only in 2012, warning of complications from decreased absorption of calcium when using antacid medications. A second warning was recently issued about decreased absorption of magnesium from the use of antacids. Now, a new study affirms that vitamin B_{12} deficiencies are increasingly common with this same group of medications. These warnings are not new information about what happens when HCl levels are suppressed, but basic knowledge about the role of HCl and the absorption of nutrients. Low levels of hydrochloric acid will lead to decreased absorption of protein, iron, iodine, B_{12}, folic acid, calcium, magnesium, zinc, and other vitamins and minerals. The loss of absorption of these nutrients will create widespread effects on health throughout the body and cause years of suffering, advanced aging, and death.

Protein

Proteins are one of the basic building blocks of the body. They make up the DNA and RNA that regulate the human genetic code and determine how everything functions in the body. Enzymes, which facilitate all reactions, are based on protein. Tissue repair and growth depend on protein. Blood sugar control depends on protein. Basic cell scaffolding is based on proteins. Proteins are critical to life and health. The breakdown and absorption of protein depends on proper levels of hydrochloric acid. Otherwise, the body cannot create pepsin, which is necessary to begin breaking down the proteins or to stimulate the release of the pancreatic enzymes necessary to complete the process—that is, breaking down the protein into its basic components: amino acids. Without amino acids for absorption, the functions associated with proteins will be lost.

Iron

Without iron to carry the oxygen to all the cells of the body, a person cannot expect to get better from anything. The importance of iron to all living organisms cannot be understated. Iron combines with proteins to form the hemoglobin that red blood cells use to carry oxygen to all cells and tissues. Iron is a part of every cell. Iron also plays a role in the formation of hydrochloric acid. Without iron, there may be no HCl, and without HCl, there may be no iron absorption. It can be a vicious cycle to break.

Iron combines with proteins to form the enzymes the body needs. An iron deficiency can affect brain function, cause fatigue, affect immunity, delay development in children, and lead to irritability and restless leg syndrome. It is an essential nutrient for health and vitality.

Iodine

Iodine is a key ingredient for thyroid function, which in turn affects almost all cells via the hormones produced by the thyroid gland. Iodine is necessary for cellular metabolism and the process of converting food to energy. Iodine also plays a role in brain and bone development. Symptoms of iodine deficiency include fatigue, cold hands and feet, hair loss, constipation, weight gain, depression, infertility, and hormonal imbalances. Since iodine can have a limiting effect on the growth of fungal candida, it makes sense that candida would create some way to decrease the absorption and presence of iodine in the body, just as it does with *Lactobacillus* bacteria and other cells and functions.

Vitamin B$_{12}$

Like other essential nutrients that are lost when HCl levels are low, vitamin B$_{12}$ is responsible for many functions in the cells and tissues. It plays a major role in the function of the nervous system, and a deficiency is frequently associated with depression, anxiety, dementia, Alzheimer's disease, moodiness, and memory loss. This vitamin plays a role in the formation of the cells and tissues of the nervous system, assists with cellular DNA, helps reduce inflammation, and is a cofactor in hundreds of reactions.

In food, vitamin B$_{12}$ is combined with proteins that require HCl in order to be separated, after which it combines with the intrinsic factor protein to be absorbed. Vitamin B$_{12}$ is essential for the function of other nutrients like folic acid and vitamin B_6. One of the main problems associated with decreased levels of B_{12} is pernicious anemia, when the body can't make enough red blood cells. In this case, the vitamin deficiency relates to a lack of the intrinsic factor protein as a result of low hydrochloric acid levels. Vitamin B_{12} deficiencies increase the risk of stomach cancer and may be a key factor in gastritis and ulcers.

Folic Acid

Folic acid, also known as vitamin B_9, and vitamin B_{12} are often considered an essential pair. Like vitamin B_{12}, folic acid deficiencies can affect DNA synthesis and create a form of anemia known as megaloblastic anemia, which is marked by underproduction of red blood cells.

ESSENTIAL

During pregnancy, folic acid helps prevent neural tube defects that affect the baby's brain or spine. The baby's brain and spine form around days 21–28. As a result, supplementing with folic acid should begin before pregnancy, since most women don't find out they're pregnant until days 42–56.

Most people are familiar with folic acid's role in preventing birth defects, which is why most foods are fortified with folic acid. It is highly recommended during pregnancy for the same reason as well. Deficiencies are rare, but symptoms may include fatigue, lightheadedness, weight loss, low libido, and loss of appetite. If a deficiency of folic acid is present, it's usually been in process for a while.

The Minerals

Calcium and magnesium are responsible for more than 500 reactions in the body. Decreased calcium absorption is commonly associated with bone loss and an increased risk of fractures, but that is just one example of how important this nutrient is to the function of all cells. Every cell requires calcium. It helps regulate the movement of fluids and nutrients in and out of the cell. Muscular contraction and relaxation, as well as nerve function and transmission, require calcium.

Calcium and magnesium are another example of a nutrient dynamic duo. Magnesium helps move calcium in and out of cells and helps ensure the ongoing reproduction of cells and life by synthesizing DNA, RNA, and the creation of energy. This mineral is a major factor in blood sugar regulation and reduction of inflammation. Candida can increase blood sugar levels and inflammation through a magnesium deficiency. These two imbalances then help increase candida overgrowth. Signs of magnesium deficiency include muscle cramps, anxiety, insomnia, irregular heartbeat, and irritability.

Zinc is another key mineral that is lost with low levels of hydrochloric acid. Zinc plays a vital role in reproduction and immune function. By lowering zinc levels, candida helps weaken an effective immune response. Signs of zinc deficiency include frequent colds, loss of appetite, delayed growth, delayed wound healing, and hair loss.

Medications

A recent study entitled "Diagnosis of Small Intestinal Bacterial Overgrowth: Does Glucose Breath Testing Measure Up?" found that 60 percent of patients taking antacid medications, such as proton-pump inhibitors (Prilosec, AcipHex, Protonix, and Nexium), had fungal overgrowth of the small intestine. Another class of antacid medications known as H2 antagonists (Tagamet, Zantac, and Ranitidine) would likely produce the same results. Antibiotic-resistant strains of bacteria were also present. Both findings point to the lasting effects of antibiotics and the risk of antacid medications.

FACT

Antacid medications have been linked to the increased risk of life-threatening *Clostridium difficile* infections. Patients on antacid medications are more susceptible to infections. One hospital reported that 75 percent of patients with *C. difficile* were on antacid medications. Each year more than 330,000 people are hospitalized with *C. difficile*; 9 percent of these hospitalizations end in death, according to the Agency for Healthcare Research and Quality.

Prolonged use of antacid medications is associated with excessive levels of the hormone gastrin in the blood, which causes hypersecretion of HCL and has been found to lead to stomach cancers. Taking antacid medications has also been shown to destroy the stomach lining. From playing a role in fungal overgrowth to cancer, widespread nutrient deficiencies, and destruction of the stomach lining, antacid medications create huge liabilities for the human body.

Testing for Hydrochloric Acid

Three approaches are used to determine hydrochloric acid levels in the stomach. In the Heidelberg pH Test, the patient swallows a small capsule and then drinks a highly alkaline solution. The capsule transmits signals from the stomach where it measures the pH of the acids present. The test is considered to be highly reliable and costs a few hundred dollars.

In the second test, which can be done at home, the patient drinks a mixture of baking soda and water. Then the individual must time how long it takes him to belch; the time limit is five minutes. A quick burp indicates adequate levels of HCl, whereas one that occurs after two minutes indicates lower levels. It's obviously not as scientific as the Heidelberg test, but appears to be just as reliable overall.

The third method is a functional assessment, based on the answer to the following question: "If you eat a steak dinner with potatoes, how long before you're hungry again?" People with low HCl levels will be full for hours because the deficiency leads to an inability to process high-protein meals.

Treatment

The link between fungal candida and low HCl levels means that a candida diet is a good way to treat these imbalances safely and effectively. Many people with skin problems like eczema and psoriasis have found that HCl supplementation helps alleviate their symptoms. These supplements are usually supplied as Betaine HCl with Pepsin.

To determine how much hydrochloric acid to take as a supplement, gradually increase your intake until you feel a slight sensation of warmth coming from the stomach, just below the rib cage. The typical protocol is as follows: Take one capsule with your meal on the first day. If no heat sensation is felt, increase the dosage to two capsules with each meal on the second day. If no heat sensation is felt, increase to three capsules with each meal on the third day. Keep increasing the dosage until you feel the sensation of warmth. Once you experience the sensation, your dosage may start to decrease rapidly. If just one capsule is too much, try a candida plan first and then try the hydrochloric acid, if you still need it. If you encounter any problems, consult your doctor.

QUESTION

Is there a limit to the dosage of hydrochloric acid capsules?
Some people have taken as many as twenty to thirty capsules with each meal before feeling any sensation of heat. After this, their dosage dropped with each meal until they were only taking five or six per meal. Some people with severe deficiencies may not feel anything even at these high dosages. Getting a good evaluation by a doctor can help you to determine which dosage would work best for you.

Constipation

The answer to how many bowel movements a person should have in one day, even from doctors, is one. However, the physiology textbooks used in medical schools state that a healthy normal is three to four bowel movements daily. The average person may have one per day but that is not healthy. Constipation is defined as three or fewer bowel movements in a week. So what constitutes a healthful number? Fewer than three bowel movements a day indicates an imbalance that needs to be addressed.

Causes of Constipation

Some of the conditions associated with causing constipation are low HCl levels, liver/gallbladder congestion, diabetes and blood sugar imbalances, inflammation, hypothyroidism, multiple sclerosis, antacid medications, and antibiotics. These causes are also associated with fungal candida, which is why it is very common for people with candida to have constipation as well. Candida is a cause as well as a side effect. In some instances, candida will exist as both a cause and a side effect and constipation is twice as likely to happen. Constipation causes a recycling of toxins and further impairs the body's ability to handle its cellular waste and debris.

Constipation leads to increased levels of inflammation, and inflammation drives the growth of candida. Candida further promotes inflammation leading to a breakdown of intestinal cells and more constipation. Candida is implicated in causing irritable bowel disease and the constipation that goes with it.

Obesity

Obesity is associated with many conditions such as diabetes, heart disease, dementia, multiple sclerosis, Alzheimer's disease, and cancer. Each of these conditions is driven by inflammation, and fungal candida is a pro-inflammatory microbe that has been linked to each of them as well.

ESSENTIAL

Very few people consider the financial side effect of personal health costs. Obesity costs individuals in terms of job discrimination, unequal pay scales, higher insurance premiums, lost wages from work due to sickness, personal limitations, and poor physical health. Financial side effects should be considered with all conditions.

The link between the bacterial flora of the intestinal tract and obesity is a huge area of research these days. As always, antibiotics are mentioned in these studies. Antibiotics reduce the diversity of the bacteria present, which in turn drives inflammation and obesity.

Inflammation and increased levels of toxicity lead to water retention. Decreasing the body's levels of inflammation and a whole-body detoxification can lead to significant weight loss that doesn't involve calorie restriction. People following a candida diet often lose excess body fat and water while preserving essential muscle mass and essential body fat on a normal-to-high-calorie diet.

What about Gluten Intolerance?

Gluten intolerance is usually described as an allergic response to a combination of proteins found in grains such as wheat, rye, barley, and the substances that are derived from them. However, it is more correctly a sensitivity rather than a true allergic response and may be either an inherited or acquired condition.

Gluten is responsible for causing bread to rise into fluffy loaves. The two proteins that make up gluten are gliadin and glutenin. Gliadin causes a sensitivity reaction.

Candida and gluten allergies are commonly seen together. The link is found in a protein on the surface of candida's cell wall. This protein (Hyphal wall protein, or Hwp1) is very similar to the alpha-gliadin and gamma-gliadin proteins found in gluten. These two gliadins stimulate autoimmune cell responses in celiac disease, a more severe form of gluten intolerance. Human immune system cells don't recognize the Hwp1 as separate from the intestinal cell. Instead they are seen as part of the same foreign material. From that point on, the immune system will target both substances either together or separately by producing antibodies against them.

FACT

You can screen for gluten allergies using several tests: the Anti-transglutaminase antibodies (anti-tTG, or ATA), the antigliadin antibodies (AGA), and the anti-endomysial antibodies (EMA) tests. A genetic test, the HLA-DQ2, can also indicate an inherited tendency toward celiac disease. See your doctor for testing.

The similarities between Hwp1 and gluten proteins can lead to autoimmune diseases like celiac disease in which the immune system attacks the cells of the intestine when gluten products are ingested. This autoimmune process has been implicated in a host of other inflammatory conditions and patterns throughout the body.

Long-term inflammation of the intestinal tract can also lead to malabsorption syndromes, anemia, immunosuppression, nervous system disorders, infertility, inflammatory bowel disorders, and cancer. Two good examples of increasingly common conditions related to candida and gluten sensitivities include autism and irritable bowel syndrome. Over the past several decades, the number of individuals with celiac disease, as well as with many other inflammatory and autoimmune conditions, has increased. Crohn's disease is seven times more likely in celiac or gluten-sensitive individuals. Today, the incidence of celiac disease is as high as one in every 100 individuals, or roughly more than 3 million people in the United States alone. Although this is a tremendous increase in a condition that was considered rare just a few decades ago; some believe it is understated. The diagnosis and resolution of fungal candida has been found to reduce the immune-system antibodies against gluten, leading to significant resolution of gluten allergies.

CHAPTER 7

The Candida Diet

The best dietary approach to addressing candida will help reduce inflammation, restrict easy energy sources, avoid common allergens, increase bacterial diversity, and increase the absorption of nutrients and the elimination of toxins. In short, it will be an approach that can be applied to almost any condition or imbalance within the body. Everyone will be able to benefit from this approach, regardless of whether they have candida.

The Essentials

In the late 1940s, the early years of treating candida, diet was never a consideration. The first candida diet wasn't created until the 1970s when Orian Truss, MD, developed an approach to eliminating candida. Most candida diets available today follow the guidelines he established. Unfortunately, Dr. Truss put more faith in antifungal drugs like Nystatin than in diet. However, his diet became entrenched in the 1980s with the release of two popular books on candida written by medical doctors: *The Yeast Syndrome* and *The Yeast Connection*. In later years, Dr. Truss stated that diet was an important factor in addressing candida, most likely due to the inability of drugs without diet to have much effect as studies have demonstrated.

FACT

Nystatin was developed by Elizabeth Lee Hazen and Rachel Fuller Brown in the 1950s to combat fungal infections arising from antibiotics. Its use is limited to the digestive tract, skin, and vaginal tissues, as it does not work systemically. Nystatin is named after New York State where it was developed and is also used in restoring artwork.

Following Dr. Truss's recommendations, these books focused on eliminating sugars from the diet. Sugary foods such as sweets, fruit juice, fruits, dried fruits, and alcohol, along with fermented foods like vinegars, cheeses, soy sauce, and yeast-based breads, were to be avoided. Anything made with or containing yeast was also not allowed. Simple carbohydrates such as pastas and some other processed, yeast-free grains were acceptable in limited amounts.

Over time, the candida diet has improved. Years of research and a better understanding about sugar, diet, and candida have improved upon the body of knowledge that was the basis for early diets. A candida diet can produce miraculous results and create a new state of health for millions of people.

Sugars

Sugars combine to form carbohydrates. Carbohydrates are either simple or complex, based on how many sugars join in a chain. Short chains of sugars form simple carbohydrates, such as candy, table sugar, honey, fruits, fruit juices, and syrups. Long chains of sugars create complex carbohydrates, which may have more than a thousand sugars in a chain. Complex carbohydrates include whole-grain breads, cereals, starchy vegetables, and legumes. The earliest candida diets recommended avoiding simple carbohydrates.

Through the years it has been found that complex carbohydrates like breads, pastas, and cereals actually break down quickly in the body to form simple sugars and should be avoided in the beginning of any candida diet. Complex carbohydrates such as yams, squashes, and many vegetables break down more slowly and are not as readily available as processed grains.

ESSENTIAL

The average person in America consumes 136–150 pounds of sugar a year. The average person in China consumes 15 pounds annually. Worldwide, Americans consume well over twice as much sugar as anyone else. The sugar industry predicts close to a 20 percent increase in business by 2020.

Sugars are an important fuel source for all the cells of the body. Like every other living cell, candida utilizes sugars very efficiently. Researchers from the University of Aberdeen in Scotland, an institution known for its research on candida, found that "*C. albicans* is exquisitely sensitive to glucose." The glucose was found to increase candida's ability to handle stress and make it more resistant to antifungal drugs and white blood cells. Another study found that reducing the intake of sugars and simple carbohydrates can reduce candida's ability to thrive when other cells are present. Researchers from South Africa found that candida was unable to grow alongside other bacteria when glucose supplies were limited. This finding is especially important as it helps illustrate that complete elimination of all carbohydrates is not typically required.

Glucose is a necessary requirement for many cells and tissues. The brain, for example, requires sugar to function effectively. The immune system suffers when too much or too little sugar is present. The beneficial bacteria of the body require sugar as much as any other cell. Eliminating all sugars is likely to impair health, not promote it. The only exception is when there is an issue regulating the body's blood sugar levels, such as with hypoglycemia, hyperglycemia, and diabetes. In those cases, sugar intake will need to be more tightly regulated, and following the Blood Sugar Protocol can help.

A balanced diet allows the natural sugars found in fruits, along with their fiber content, antioxidants, and minerals to continue supporting the body's energy needs and health. Most candida diets have been criticized for their removal of all carbohydrate sources, because the body needs this fuel source.

Protein and Fats

Apart from sugars, proteins and fats are good foods to consume on a candida diet. Starting your day with protein and having protein at your main meals helps keep blood sugar levels more balanced, which helps reduce excess sugars as a fuel source for candida. Fats are an excellent source of energy as well. Fats in the form of oils should be, when possible, organic and cold-pressed or virgin oils. Most fatty acids that make up the oils and fats that are consumed have antifungal properties, especially virgin coconut and extra-virgin olive oils.

Everything Is Food

Advances in science have shown that almost everything is food to candida. The organism comes well equipped with enzymes like proteases to break down proteins, lipases to break down fat, and amylases and glucosidases to break down carbohydrates.

QUESTION

If candida can live off everything, can it ever be eliminated?
Balance in the intestinal tract is the key factor that keeps candida present in its normal, harmless yeast form. Antibiotics destroy that balance. Only the excessive and problematic fungal form of candida needs to be addressed. The yeast form should always be there.

Fungal candida can exist under most conditions in the body, at varying degrees of activity, surviving off whatever nutrients are available. Research has shown that candida can survive under extremely limited food conditions, such as those that exist inside white blood cells. In fact, removing all food sources can be another trigger that causes the normal yeast form of candida to convert to its pathological, problematic fungal form. In its fungal form, it can then search and derive food from almost any tissue and cell in the body.

Fermented Foods

Fermented foods are made by allowing natural bacterial cultures and processes to predigest foods through the action of bacterial enzymes. This process can help increase the availability of nutrients in food and make them easier for the body to digest. The bacteria multiply and grow during this fermentation process and become part of the final product.

The bacteria provide additional benefits to the body, much like taking probiotics. Fermented foods, however, may present problems initially when following a candida diet, and should be avoided for the first eight weeks. Fermented foods have varying levels of histamine, a substance that plays a role in allergic responses and inflammation, both of which are increased during candida infections. The imbalance in the composition of bacterial flora found after antibiotic use and candida's regulatory influence can increase the levels of histamine normally present in the intestinal tract.

Candida creates an immune response that plays a role in allergic reactions. Extra histamine will exacerbate this response and drive allergies and inflammation. Fermented foods can contain residues of sugars and alcohol that may facilitate fungal candida growth.

Candida promotes inflammation by increasing the production of prostaglandins, a fatty substance that increases inflammation. Histamine can also increase prostaglandins and with candida has been shown to synergistically increase prostaglandin levels. Increased levels of prostaglandins will also enhance the growth and formation of fungal candida.

Once normal levels of candida in its yeast form have been established, and the bacterial flora, immune system, and cellular responses have been balanced, then fermented foods are highly recommended.

Antifungals

Using an antifungal is highly recommended during a candida diet. Without antifungals, the diet may slow candida but won't eliminate it. Try a good fatty acid like undecenoic acid. Other fatty acids like caprylic acid can be useful but are less effective. Medications pose obvious health risks and create stronger antifungal-resistant strains. Medications also further suppress the immune system and lead to rebound candida infections.

Herbs also inhibit candida but do not eliminate it. The ineffectiveness of herbs alone has led some people to rotate antifungal herbs, rationalizing that candida develops resistance to the herbs if used continuously. What they are observing is the limited usefulness of herbs. When they use a new herb, they may see some effects, but the problem remains. Resistance is only created by medications, which tend to kill candida, and therefore candida adapts and the medications are no longer effective.

Inflammation

Correcting fungal candida requires simultaneously correcting its environment, as they are intricately linked. Foods play an important role in this process. Due to candida's ability to drive inflammation, a candida diet needs to be an anti-inflammatory diet as well.

In addition to the easy fuel sources that candida feeds upon, avoid common allergens, such as dairy, soy, nuts, and most grains except brown rice. Avoid fermented foods, which tend to be higher in histamine, until week 9 of the diet. Foods that are high in histamine and tyramine can instigate inflammation. These foods generally include shellfish, kefir, yogurt, dried fruit, chocolate, cocoa, vinegars, condiments, oranges, and processed, smoked, and cured meats. At first, avoid any foods that currently cause allergies or other imbalances, but you may be able to add them later when more balance is restored to your digestive system.

FACT

The acronym for the Standard American Diet is SAD. Whenever this highly inflammatory diet is introduced to other countries around the world, their rates of diabetes, heart disease, stroke, obesity, and auto-immune diseases increase dramatically.

The Power of Nature

At all levels of life, there is a natural ecosystem. The laws that govern these ecosystems appear to function in similar ways. Life is important, balance is necessary, and diversity is the key to health. Antibiotics along with fungal candida damage our internal ecosystem by destroying life, creating imbalance, and reducing diversity. Fortunately, nature provides us with many ways to counter these insults.

The microbial flora within the intestinal tract have been referred to as the densest ecosystem on the planet. Anyone who has ever spent time in a jungle can readily appreciate how dense that would have to be. The larger ecosystem contains all types of plants whose roots, stems, leaves, flowers, and fruits have been used for centuries for their many healing benefits. The study of these plants or herbs has given humans many tools for maintaining and improving health.

One of the busiest areas of scientific research is the field of epigenetics, the study of how the environment around and within humans shapes how human genes function and behave. Genes are the basic building blocks of the cells that determine how the body's cells develop and function. Factors that can produce an epigenetic effect include diet, toxins, thoughts, emotions, and stress. Processed foods tend to exert a negative impact on genes and therefore on health. Fruits and vegetables, on the other hand, especially organic versions free of pesticides, chemicals, and genetic modification, have been shown to be capable of reversing most diseases and conditions through their epigenetic effect.

Herbs have also been shown to have this effect. By increasing your intake of organic whole foods and herbs, you are helping to ensure that your body has a good supply of tools to keep it healthy. The current U.S. government recommendation for daily intake of fruits and vegetables is five servings of each, for a total of ten servings per day. In a clinical study, the daily intake of fruits and vegetables before following a candida diet was one serving. Those people following a candida diet were eating ten or more servings per day, meeting and exceeding the recommended intake. The potential health benefits of this factor alone are truly amazing.

ESSENTIAL

Pharmaceutical companies derive many of their drugs from the study of beneficial substances produced by plants and fungi. Scientists have yet to study the more than 200,000 plant species in the Amazon rainforests alone.

In nature, all plants contain a pharmacy, which can quickly produce the exact substance necessary to defend the plant from threats. If bacteria threaten a plant species or even an entire community, plants will manufacture antibiotics that prevent it from destroying them. These antibiotics have no long-term effects and are sufficient to control the bacteria without producing strains of antibiotic resistance. Humans can only dream of such abilities. In nature, the role of fungus is often to break down matter and recycle it into the soil as a rich supply of nutrients for continued plant growth. Almost all plants produce antifungal substances that prevent fungus from destroying them. This process continues until the plant dies, at which point the fungus fulfills one of its important roles in the ecosystem. Because of these antifungal properties, many plants make a welcome addition to a candida diet. Antifungal foods include garlic, onions, ginger, lemons, limes, and all oils, especially coconut and olive oil. Be sure to include them in your candida diet.

Yes Foods

During a candida diet, certain foods will help correct fungal imbalances and certain foods won't. Yes Foods have been found to work best with the diet because they are high-quality, nutritious whole foods that don't typically create or add to inflammation and allergic responses or provide an easy fuel source for candida. When used with a good antifungal, Yes Foods can produce excellent results. If any of the foods on this list already create problems for you, avoid them initially on the diet.

Some people with lifelong food allergies have seen these allergies resolve themselves while following a candida diet. Avoid problem foods at first, and after a few weeks, try them to see if they still present problems. If they continue to be problematic, wait until finishing the diet to see if the allergic responses are still present. The following list of Yes Foods is for the first eight weeks of a sixteen-week program. Beginning in week 9, certain foods will be added back every two weeks.

- All meats (except pork)
- All vegetables (includes potatoes)
- All fresh fruits (except oranges)
- Eggs
- Brown rice (long- or short-grain)
- Brown rice cereal, hot
- Tea, coffee
- Virgin or cold-pressed oils
- Seasonings

Meats

Approved meats include beef, buffalo, chicken, turkey, fish, fowl, emu, and ostrich, for those with a more exotic taste. These last two meats are more recent additions to world markets. Pork doesn't seem to work as well with the diet. Some holistic practitioners recommend against it; from a clinical perspective, their patients seem to feel worse when eating it.

Each pork cell contains a virus called porcine endogenous retrovirus (PERV). Whether this can create a problem is not known. Some studies have shown that PERV infects human cells and others have shown the opposite to be true. This may have nothing to do with the reaction observed in patients, but there does seem to be a greater increase in inflammation in people consuming pork. Part of the problem with pork may be due to overexposure to pigs raised under industrialized farming practices, where antibiotics are fed repeatedly. It is possible that free-range, grass-fed, pastured pigs would be okay, but that still may not work in people who have consumed a lifetime of factory-raised pork. For at least the first eight weeks, avoid pork. Smoked, processed, and cured meats should also be avoided during the diet. These meats have been found to have higher amounts of tyramine, histamine, and fungus, and have a greater association risk with certain cancers.

Vegetables

All vegetables are included on the candida diet. Along with fruits, these foods provide a powerful abundance of healthful benefits. Vegetables tend to have higher fiber content and are processed more slowly. Some of the complex carbohydrates found in vegetables can be a good source of sugars for the body's cells and bacteria but a poor choice for fungal candida. Complex carbohydrates are less likely to affect blood sugar levels as dramatically as simple carbohydrates. An adequate intake of carbohydrates ensures a healthy immune system and neurological function, as well as fueling the beneficial bacteria. Researchers from Australia and the United Kingdom have shown that reduced amounts of carbohydrates can alter the composition of the bacterial flora leading to an increased risk of inflammation, cell damage, leaky gut, and cancer. Obviously, carbohydrates provide benefits that are essential to health.

QUESTION

Is it safe to avoid all fruits and sweet vegetables during a candida diet?
Over the course of several months, there may be no harm done. There are definitely many benefits to eating such foods. On the other hand, the North American Inuit people have an excellent history of health, and they eat few, if any, fruits and vegetables. Their life expectancy, however, is less than average.

Potatoes can be problematic for people with blood sugar issues. If eating potatoes appears to increase your blood sugar imbalances, avoid them. Yams and sweet potatoes do not produce the same effect.

ESSENTIAL

The abundance of vegetables and fruits on a candida diet provides vegetarians and vegans with an equal opportunity to address fungal candida.

Fruits

The original candida diets gave fruits a bad name. Staunch adherents to the original format are missing the wonderful benefits that fruits provide, and they may be placing themselves at risk by reducing all sources of sugar. Fruits are an excellent way to improve and maintain the health of all the body's systems, organs, tissues, and cells.

Most people following a candida diet exceed the recommended dietary intake of fruits and vegetables. One fruit that appears to be an exception is oranges. Overconsumption of oranges that have been sprayed with pesticides and fungicides has led to an allergic response that is difficult to correct. Many mothers refuse to give their children orange juice or oranges when they have a cold because the oranges increase the amount of mucus produced. The body's allergic response to the high levels of tyramine and histamine in oranges increases the amounts of mucus present.

Excess mucus can make it more difficult to correct fungal candida imbalances and can interfere with the absorption of nutrients and elimination of toxins. Other citrus fruits such as grapefruit, lemon, lime, and pineapple also have histamines and tyramines present. These fruits are less likely to create an excess mucus response, because there is significantly less exposure to them than to oranges.

Eggs

Eggs are a complete source of protein and contain many nutrients. Whether you eat them over-easy, hard-boiled, or scrambled, eggs work well with a candida diet. Some people are concerned that eating too many eggs will lead to heart disease or stroke, but studies show that this is not a valid concern. A paper published in the *British Medical Journal* looked at more than a dozen studies on eggs and found no correlation. Earlier studies that examined the risk of eggs and high cholesterol were found to have serious design flaws with exaggerated results. The cholesterol contained in egg yolks is an excellent source of fat and other nutrients. Most health practitioners suggest eating eggs with the yolks still runny to avoid overcooking and oxidation of the cholesterol in the yolk. A study from the Harvard School of Public Health showed that moderate egg consumption of up to one egg per day was not associated with any increased risk of heart disease. Whichever way you like your eggs appears to be okay as long as you eat them.

Brown Rice

Brown rice is a good source of fiber and contains other nutrients that have been shown to have beneficial effects. Researchers at Harvard University found that, when compared to white rice, consumption of brown rice led to a lower risk of diabetes. Brown rice is the whole-grain version with the bran and germ layers intact; white rice, on the other hand, has the bran and germ removed along with many of the nutrients. A Temple University study found that brown rice was associated with cardiovascular benefits that were missing with white rice.

Sweating

Some studies have found that hot baths and saunas are beneficial and pose no risks to people with hypertension, congestive heart failure, and heart disease when properly medicated. In the study titled "Health effects and risks of sauna bathing," researchers in Finland stated, "no adverse effects during pregnancy were found." The benefits and safety of saunas and hot baths are found in numerous studies, validating what many cultures have practiced for centuries.

Sweating should be an integral part of a candida diet. Any imbalance involving fungal candida tends to represent an imbalance in overall health. The body is a sponge in its environment, soaking up chemicals, heavy metals, and other toxins. Water-soluble toxins are quickly eliminated, but fat-soluble toxins bind themselves to fat stores. This binding can help protect the organs and tissues, but greater levels of fat eventually lead to greater levels of inflammation and predisposition to diabetes and other diseases. In very thin people, there is a greater risk of those toxins depositing within their vital organs, leading to a quicker onset of disease, deterioration, and advanced aging.

FACT

Researchers at the University of Alberta found that sweat contained metals and chemicals not found in urine and blood, and that "many toxic elements appeared to be preferentially excreted through sweat."

More than 140,000 chemicals are added to the environment every year. Each year, anywhere from 2,000 to 4,000 new chemicals are added to the list of chemicals that enter the environment. Toxic loads vary depending on your environment. Living in a major city can greatly increase the toxic burden. People in many Chinese cities face some of the worst conditions known on the planet with air pollution levels constantly exceeding dangerous levels. A good day in Beijing might equal the worst day in Los Angeles.

Babies are being born with levels of toxins that were never known before. "Scientific fact" once held that babies were protected from chemicals and toxins by the placenta and umbilical cord. Unfortunately, this is not true, and babies are being born with hundreds of toxins already in their bodies. Of the 140,000+ chemicals that are documented, very few have been studied for their effects on humans. Some suppress the immune system, some cause hormonal disruption, some cause cancer, and some cause neurological diseases. Beyond that, very little is known about them.

Most of these chemicals stimulate the same immune response that favors the growth of fungal candida. Those chemicals and heavy metals that suppress the immune system also tend to promote the growth of candida. One of the well-known heavy metals in this area is the mercury found in silver amalgam dental fillings. Some people with severe immune suppression due to mercury have found it difficult to correct fungal candida imbalances. Candida has been shown to possess an ability to transform the nontoxic elemental form of mercury to its methyl form, which is toxic to human cells and bacteria. Candida most likely uses this ability to further its growth and spread throughout the body.

Mercury increases levels of inflammation in the body and can disrupt the blood-brain barrier and cause inflammation of the brain. Many chemicals mimic the effect of estrogens, which can suppress immune responses that are the most effective against candida. Sweating helps increase the body's metabolic rate and detoxify the tissues; it is effective for helping release heavy metals. The elimination of chemicals and heavy metals and other waste products can help to reduce inflammation and the immune imbalances that go with it.

While doing a candida diet, sweating six days a week, ten minutes a day, during a sixteen-week diet with fatty acid antifungals has been the most beneficial. Longer sessions can assist the body in eliminating more toxins. Some people have even tried two sessions daily. Although this method doesn't correct fungal candida any faster it can help the body in other ways.

This kind of sweating is not accomplished through exercise; muscular contraction during exercise can interfere with clearing toxins effectively. The best forms of sweating are in a sauna, hot bath, hot tub, or steam rooms. Bikram, or hot, yoga has also been found to work, as the ambient temperature is around 105°F. You can also buy large or small sauna units for home and personal use. Small personal saunas that are very effective cost around $200. These small portable saunas enjoyed popularity during the 1950s and 1960s due to the increased interest in the benefits of sweating and detoxification at that time, but they fell out of use after that. Portable saunas have since regained their popularity and are being used more and more in homes once again.

QUESTION

Can women take a hot bath during their menstrual cycle?
Most women find that hot baths during their menstrual cycle are soothing and can help relieve cramping. Hot baths can also help reduce stress and anxiety. Harsh soaps or gels may cause irritation, but a little bubble bath may be just fine. Saunas or steam rooms can be good alternatives during these days.

It's a good practice to drink plenty of purified water while sweating. If you feel faint when initially beginning a sweating protocol, place a cold washcloth across the back of your neck and drink cold water to help reduce the symptoms. If you feel dizzy, don't attempt to stand until you feel better. If you're not used to sweating, it can take a session or two for your body to adapt. Don't rush it. In no time, you'll be extending your sweating sessions and enjoying your time alone.

In addition, taking a good trace mineral product, such as Trace Minerals ConcenTrace, can offset deficiencies. Many busy people often find that taking time out to sweat allows them to rest, recuperate, and enjoy a few moments of well-deserved peace. They soon begin looking forward to their sweating sessions and a little time for themselves. These sessions are a good time to read, meditate, or just relax and free the mind.

How Long Does It Take?

A successful dietary approach to correcting fungal candida levels, boosting the immune system response against candida, and restoring normal tissue flora usually requires about sixteen weeks. It takes a commitment to being healthy to make it happen.

ESSENTIAL

There's always going to be a party, wedding, anniversary, birthday, vacation, or celebration to tempt you away from your diet. Don't give in!

During the first eight weeks, follow the Yes and No Foods lists. Beginning in week 9, you can start adding back certain foods every two weeks until the end of the sixteen weeks. Be sure to take a supplement to boost the immune system (such as vitamin C or echinacea) while you are on the plan. Also be sure to include a good fatty acid antifungal like undecenoic acid during the first eight weeks. The dosage should be at 5 3x/day, which equals 250 mg, three times a day for a daily total of 750 mg, and can be taken all the way through the plan. Some people choose to take a maintenance dosage of five capsules once a day after week 8. Taking higher doses doesn't appear to speed the process. Probiotics should be started in week 7 and taken until the end. Starting probiotics in week 7 enables the candida in the intestinal tract to be balanced first to make room for the beneficial bacteria to grow and implant into the intestinal flora. Since candida prevents many species of certain bacteria from growing back in the body after antibiotic use, correcting fungal candida first is a must. Waiting until week 7 to add probiotics also allows time to balance immune-system responses that can ensure that candida can't return in its fungal form. Once these responses have been established, probiotics help ensure that these responses remain intact.

Some people benefit by continuing the diet beyond the sixteen-week period to allow their body to eliminate more toxins and repair important pathways that may have been affected by years of inflammation and deterioration. Balancing the immune system can take longer if toxins have built up in the tissue for years. Many symptoms can improve quickly on a candida diet. Some may take longer, which can represent a more complex issue. Allow your body time to heal. If you extend the diet and still find that a symptom hasn't resolved, look into other health measures. Chemicals and heavy metals may play a role, and while many of these can be eliminated on this diet, you may need a specific heavy-metal detox to eliminate problematic heavy metals and chemicals buried deeper in the body more effectively. Not everything is caused by candida. This attitude can lead to months and years of frustration. Consult a holistic practitioner, preferably one with years of experience in helping others heal.

CHAPTER 8

Cooking on the Diet

Preparing meals and snacks for a candida diet plan can be easy, fun, and cathartic. The meals you eat can be as complicated or as easy as you wish, while creating and sharing your recipes can be inspirational and rewarding. On this diet, food becomes medicine and the kitchen cabinet becomes the medicine cabinet.

Preparation, Preparation, Preparation

Change can be challenging, especially when it comes to changing your dietary habits. Preparation is probably the best way to achieve success and ensure that you're less likely to stumble on the diet. If you have everything that you need, you won't fall into old habits. Stock up on foods that you know are okay and give away the foods that you don't need. Unless you live with people who are not following the diet, there's no reason to keep temptation within arm's reach.

Time

Get up early and spend thirty to forty-five minutes preparing meals and snacks for your day. Some people do this at night so that they're ready to go in the morning. Each person's lifestyle will determine what works best. Parents often have to prepare their family's meals first and then their own. Eating a whole foods–based diet is good for everyone, so you can base the majority of what is served in the house on your dietary plan.

Prepare foods that work for you and let your family add the condiments or sauces at the table. You can prepare certain foods and then do something else, like the ten minutes of daily sweating. For example, throw four to six yams in the oven to bake while you take a hot bath. A large roast can take an hour or more depending on its weight.

Placing food in a slow cooker early in the morning or late at night can help as well. A slow cooker usually has two settings: low and high. The low setting cooks foods over eight to ten hours. The high setting is for foods that require two to three hours. You can go to work and when you come home, dinner will be ready.

FACT

The original slow cooker, the Crock-Pot, was developed in 1971 and quickly became a household name. Originally designed to cook beans, it was modified to cook meat by the Rival Company. Many imitators quickly flooded the market, but few remain today. The Sunbeam Corporation now owns the Crock-Pot brand.

Grocery List

Make a special shopping list so that you know exactly what foods fit your new dietary lifestyle. You're less likely to wander down the aisles of No Foods when you know there's nothing there for you. A whole foods–based lifestyle means you'll be shopping around the outside edges of the grocery store where the healthiest, anti-inflammatory foods are usually located.

Broths and Stocks

Making broths and stocks is an excellent way to extract as many nutrients as possible from a variety of foods. The two terms are used interchangeably in most recipes. Slow cookers are a good way to prepare stocks, but many cooks simmer the ingredients in a big pot on the stove.

Start by adding your ingredients to a pot of cold water and then heating everything on very low heat or on the simmer setting. The bones of meats can be a powerhouse of nutrients that help heal years of chronic intestinal inflammation or help keep your skin looking younger and wrinkle-free. Bone-broth recipes usually call for slowly cooking the bones for one to two days. Marrow bones are available at most grocery stores and butcher shops. The gelatin created by bone broths helps heal leaky gut, arthritis, irritable bowel syndrome, liver toxicity, colic, allergies, and mineral deficiencies. It can be an excellent first food for babies who are weaning. Including broths in your diet will heal and support your body in many ways.

Snacks

Make sure that you have plenty of snacks on hand while on the diet. Fresh vegetables and fruits, if you can eat them, are excellent snacks. Plain rice cakes also work very well. Top them off with sliced avocado or dip them in almond oil. Try topping a rice cake with slices of banana. Rice cakes also make an excellent substitute for popcorn at the movies.

Protein is another excellent snack. You can roll up sliced avocado and tomato in thin slices of beef, buffalo, or turkey. Experiment with all kinds of vegetables. Asparagus, mint or basil leaves, lettuce, and cucumbers are excellent roll-up ingredients. Another option is to use lettuce leaves for the outside of the roll-up. Celery cut up into 3-inch sections makes a good snack that's easy to prepare and take with you, and it doesn't spoil. It also works well with the Blood Sugar Protocol.

Juicing

Juicing is a great way to enjoy nutrients from vegetables. With the correct juicer, you can extract live enzymes and nutrients from vegetables in a form that is easier for the body to absorb and use. A powerful blender like the Vitamix won't extract as many nutrients as a cold-press juicer, but it does allow you to obtain a good source of fiber that helps feed the bacteria of the colon. Limit your juices to green vegetable juices, ginger, turmeric, and other veggies that aren't sweet. Avoid fruit juice and sweet vegetable juices—such as carrots, tomatoes, beets, potatoes—for at least the first eight weeks.

Juicers and Blenders

Juicers and blenders are great for green juices and smoothies, as well as for hot drinks. Closed-case, crush-press juicers, also known as masticating or cold-press juicers, extract and preserve nutrients very well. Typical brands include Green Star, Bella, Hurom, Samson, and Omega. These juicers can cost from $300 to $500 and typically have ten-year warranties. To help preserve the nutrients, these juicers gently crush the food instead of whirling it like centrifugal juicers. This process creates higher amounts of oxygen, which can rapidly destroy the nutrients in the food and not produce as much juice. The Norwalk Juicer, developed in 1934, is often considered the best cold-press juicer. Its two-step process—grinding and pressing—is credited with extracting a higher amount of nutrients and enzymes than other good juicers on the market. The pressing step enables greater nutrient and enzyme extraction from the juices. The Norwalk's main drawback is its price tag: about $2,500. If the price is no issue and you're really into juicing, then this may be the juicer for you.

Centrifugal juicers include the Breville, Omega, Fusion, and Bella. Some companies make both kids of juicers, so make sure that you know which type you want to purchase. The price tag will be a good indicator, as centrifugal juicers are typically less expensive.

QUESTION

Do you have to purchase a cold-press juicer or will a centrifugal juicer work as well?
The advantage of the cold-press juicer is the higher quality of the juice extracted, where the nutrients are better preserved. Centrifugal juicers have worked just as effectively for many people who use juices as part of an anticancer protocol or for other health reasons. Preference and cost will be your determining factors.

Mini handheld mixers come with and without cords and are great for mixing up drinks with spices and oils. Cordless versions like the Norpro are inexpensive and portable. The Aero Latte frother is a similar mixer. Dynamic makes more powerful, corded miniblenders that are much more expensive, costing close to $500. The power, however, leads to greater levels of oxygenation and nutrient loss if used with vegetable juices. Do not add ice to your juices; the ice can affect digestion and absorption of nutrients.

Spread the Word

Let your friends know that you are following a candida diet and ask for their support. Even if you're concerned about what they'll think, don't be afraid to tell them. You're more likely to get their support if you're honest. It lets them know how much you respect what they think, which is a nice compliment that will almost always be returned with kindness.

Many people are surprised not only by how well their friends respond, but also by the amount of interest they express. People who follow a candida diet plan become examples and leaders for their friends and family. The healthy changes that they see taking place with you will be an inspiration. Leading by example is the best way to assist others. If nothing else, it ensures that you are as healthy as possible.

Nature's Gifts

Nature has blessed us with a vast array of fruits and vegetables that both nourish and protect us. Incorporating known "power" foods into your diet can produce additional benefits in many ways. A good key to follow is color. The more colorful your food selection, the healthier it will be for you. The color in many foods is due to a group of plant pigments known as carotenoids that act as antioxidants. They have produced excellent research results in studies on cancer and other diseases. Turn your dinner plate into a rainbow of colors and enjoy the foods' beauty and healthful benefits. Take the opportunity to have your own garden or plant some herbs in your flower boxes. The best foods are homegrown and picked fresh.

FACT

More than 600 known carotenoids are found in nature, although only a few of their benefits are well known and researched. Two groups in the carotenoid family are carotenes and xanthophylls. Beta-carotene is the best known carotenoid and readily converts to vitamin A in the body. Lutein and zeaxanthin are two popular xanthophylls with known health benefits for the eyes.

Plants are also an excellent source of minerals, antioxidants, fibers, and other amazing nutrients. A study done by National Geographic, called the Blue Zone Study, found that a common factor in people who lived to 100 and older was a diet that was 80 percent plant-based. Eating a diverse variety of plants provides an abundance of nutrients that support a healthy internal ecosystem. Appendix B has an in-depth list of the foods you can turn to for these incredible nutrients.

Keeping It Simple

This book contains 150 recipes for those creative types who like to explore a wide variety of menu choices. Others who do better with simple choices and don't mind repetition will find that the candida diet plan can work equally as well for them. Throwing some eggs, tomatoes, brown rice, avocado, and beef in a pan for a morning scramble doesn't take a lot of skill and can be done very quickly. Preparing some hard-boiled eggs by the dozen and grabbing them as a snack or using a few as a meal can work well. Cooking large pots of foods can make it easier to stay on a candida diet. Cook enough brown rice for the week and use it as needed. Cook large pots of vegetables in a slow cooker and add them to the brown rice and other dishes throughout the week. Reheating the food takes a few minutes.

Does microwaving food destroy the nutrients?
Heating food can lower the nutrient content and destroy the enzymes present. Some studies have compared the microwave to boiling and cooking and found minor differences in nutrient content among the different types of heating methods. Until more is known, using the recommended low settings may be best if you can't give up your microwave.

It is healthier to cook on a stove or in the oven. Like tending a garden, cooking in this way allows your creative processes and mindfulness to be present. Foods cooked in the microwave may present unnecessary health risks and tend to magnify and sustain a feeling of being rushed.

Dining Out

Dining out is generally much easier on a candida diet plan than with other types of dietary protocols. Apart from fast-food restaurants, most restaurants serve the whole foods that form the foundation of the diet. With more and more people experiencing dietary restrictions for health reasons or having allergic reactions to certain foods, restaurants have relaxed their policies and now serve their customers' interests with more flexibility than years ago.

Bragg Liquid Aminos can be a good substitute for many sauces, and the small bottle fits nicely into a purse or bag. It's delicious on meats and veggies. It's also non-GMO and kosher!

Restaurants will withhold sauces from meals since they are usually added in the last step of preparation. Meats and vegetables can all be served without sauces, dressings, and condiments. Remember that sugar is a hidden ingredient in many sauces. So if you're unsure, ask to have the sauce served on the side.

Don't worry about oils when dining out. It's hard to control everything when it comes to foods and restaurants. Save the cold-pressed oils for home or carry a small bottle with you. Marinades will not usually be an issue either, but if you do eat at a restaurant frequently and always ask for marinated dishes, chances are you're addressing a sugar craving and you may want to order something without a marinade.

As a rule, if you're ever in doubt about something on the menu, don't order it. Restaurants will use canned sauces that have sugars in them, but the restaurant itself might not add extra sugar to a dish. If you ask the waitstaff if there is any sugar added to the meal, he or she may say no, not knowing about sugar in canned sauces. Don't feel rushed when dining out and ask a few simple questions to keep yourself on track. It should be easy enough to find restaurants that work for you.

When you reach week 7 of the plan and need to take probiotics twenty to thirty minutes before a meal, it's nice to know that the probiotics travel well outside the refrigerator. Carry them in your car, purse, or bag and take them just before going into the restaurant.

Genetically Modified Organisms in the Kitchen?

Genetically modified organisms (GMOs) are a hot topic these days. However, escalating levels of health consciousness and an increasing interest in knowing more about how food is produced and where it comes from have created a growing backlash against their use. Studies have shown that some of the altered products, mainly food, can transmit antibiotic-resistant genes without the knowledge of the consumer. Antibiotic use in livestock and humans, however, poses a much greater threat in terms of transferring antibiotic resistance.

The results are not in on the impact of GMOs on human health. A small effect in one person may have greater impact in another. Pre-existing conditions always play a role. Currently, the impact of GMOs on the environment appears to be the bigger threat.

Fortunately, GMOs are currently limited to just a few foods that for the most part aren't on the candida diet plan. Choosing organic foods is the best way to ensure that GMOs aren't present. If you stick with whole foods, and buy organic whenever possible, you'll have a better chance of avoiding GMOs until more is known about their effects.

CHAPTER 9

Breakfast Ideas

Huevos Rancheros Without Tortillas
116

Egg Lasagna
117

Brown Rice Frittata
118

Egg and Spinach Bake
118

Farmers' Scrambler
119

Sunrise Scrambler
120

South of the Border Scrambler
120

Huevos Rancheros Without Tortillas

This is a classic dish from South of the Border. In place of tortillas, try using plain brown rice cakes. It gives the meal a nice crunch!

INGREDIENTS | SERVES 2

2 medium tomatoes, peeled and coarsely chopped

2 small shallots, coarsely chopped

3 tablespoons olive oil

½ teaspoon coarse salt, plus more for seasoning

2 large eggs (organic free-range preferred)

Freshly ground pepper, to taste

Fresh cilantro leaves, for garnish

1 jalapeño pepper, seeded and finely chopped, for garnish

Top It Off with an Avocado

Make your Huevos Rancheros a complete, protein-full breakfast by serving half an avocado on top. Avocados are a delicious, creamy, healthful, complete source of protein, containing 67 percent monosaturated fats, which support cardiovascular health. Not only are avocados good for you, they'll give your dish a gourmet look.

1. Chop the tomatoes and shallots finely, or put them in a blender to make a chunky salsa.

2. Heat 2 tablespoons of oil in a nonstick pan over medium heat.

3. Add the chopped tomatoes and shallots and season with the salt. Cover the pan with a lid and let cook at medium heat, stirring occasionally, about 5 minutes, until the shallots are limp. Set aside.

4. Heat the remaining tablespoon of oil in a medium nonstick skillet over medium.

5. Crack the eggs into the skillet and cook sunny-side up (until the whites are set and the yolks are still soft), about 2 minutes. If you prefer the yolks fully cooked, cook the eggs a little longer with the lid on.

6. Slide each egg onto a plate. Pour the cooked sauce onto the eggs so that the sauce covers the entire egg.

7. Season with salt and pepper, and place the cilantro and jalapeño on top for garnish.

Egg Lasagna

This is an Italian variation on an American classic! Add even more spices and herbs like basil, thyme, garlic, and oregano to take advantage of Italy's best-known healing spices.

INGREDIENTS | SERVES 2

3 eggs (organic free-range preferred)

3 tablespoons water

1 cup chopped spinach

2 black olives, sliced

2 cups candida-approved tomato sauce or salsa (save half for topping)

Make Your Own Tomato Sauce

Canned tomatoes are not allowed until week 9 on the candida diet. You can make your own simple and delicious sauce by chopping 4 tomatoes, sautéing them in 2 tablespoons olive oil, 1 tablespoon dried basil, 1 tablespoon dried oregano, ½ clove garlic, and salt and pepper to taste. Cook all the ingredients in a medium saucepan over medium heat until the tomatoes are fully cooked and the sauce has a chunky texture.

1. Preheat the oven to 375°F.

2. In a small bowl, beat the eggs and water. Pour into an oiled 10"–15" omelet pan and fry the eggs over medium heat for 3–5 minutes.

3. Slide the flat omelet onto a large, rimmed 9" × 13" cookie sheet.

4. In a medium bowl, mix the remainder of the ingredients for the filling.

5. Spread the filling on half of the omelet. Roll the omelet over. Cover the roll with the remaining tomato sauce.

6. Bake for 20 minutes.

Brown Rice Frittata

Slowly cooking or even baking this combination at 450°F for 20 minutes can result in a fluffier omelet-style breakfast meal.

INGREDIENTS | SERVES 3

6 eggs (organic free-range preferred)
1 cup brown rice, cooked
1 clove garlic
1 cup vegetables of your choosing

1. Beat the eggs, adding the rice, garlic, and vegetables.

2. Scramble the mixture in a nonstick omelet pan over low-medium heat, for 3–5 minutes.

3. Serve and enjoy.

Make It a Green Frittata

Put 1 cup of raw broccoli in a food processor and process until the broccoli is finely chopped. Mix with the eggs. Broccoli will give your omelet an attractive green color and will help bind the brown rice.

Egg and Spinach Bake

This is a fast, easy recipe to make. Starting your morning with protein helps keep your blood sugar balanced throughout the day.

INGREDIENTS | SERVES 3

3 eggs (organic free-range preferred)
2 tablespoons virgin coconut oil
1 pound chopped spinach

1. Preheat the oven to 325°F. In a medium bowl, whip the eggs until fluffy.

2. Prepare a medium-size casserole dish by oiling it with the virgin coconut oil. Add the eggs to the dish, and then add the spinach. Fold gently to combine.

3. Bake in the preheated oven for 25–30 minutes.

Make It a Full Dinner

You can make this dish a complete dinner by adding ground beef, chicken, or turkey. Start by cooking half a pound of the protein of your choice, seasoned with your favorite spices. Let the cooked meat cool down before adding it to the egg-and-spinach mixture.

Farmers' Scrambler

Farmers understand that a healthy breakfast is the best way to prepare for a long day of work. Starting strong will help you finish strong.

INGREDIENTS | SERVES 6

2 cups diced Russet potatoes

3 tablespoons olive oil

½ cup sliced mushrooms

¼ cup chopped red bell peppers

¼ cup chopped red onions

8 eggs (organic free-range preferred)

¼ teaspoon salt

¼ teaspoon black pepper

Give It a French Touch

Add 1 tablespoon of the classic French herb blend, herbes de Provence, to give your scrambler a little something extra. This blend includes savory, marjoram, rosemary, thyme, oregano, and, in some cases, lavender. You can find this herb mixture in most supermarkets.

1. In a medium sauté pan, sauté the diced potatoes in olive oil over medium until tender, about 8–10 minutes.

2. In a separate medium sauté pan, add the sliced mushrooms, peppers, and onions and sauté over medium heat for 5 minutes.

3. Combine the contents of both pans in one large pan.

4. Beat the eggs in a medium bowl. Add them to the vegetable mix, and cook over medium heat for 3 minutes.

5. Season with salt and black pepper.

Sunrise Scrambler

The modern process of making breakfast the biggest meal of the day comes from Chinese medicinal and historical tradition. The Chinese found that the stomach was the organ with the highest activity between 7:00 and 9:00 A.M.

INGREDIENTS | SERVES 2

½ pound ground beef
½ cup chopped mushrooms
6 eggs (organic free-range preferred)
½ cup tomatoes, diced

A Fun and Colorful Twist

Give this recipe a fun and tasty twist by adding colorful red, yellow, and green bell peppers. Chop up a quarter of each pepper, sauté them with the mushrooms, and season the mixture with salt and pepper. If you want a little heat, add ½ jalapeño.

1. In a large frying pan over medium heat, cook the ground beef for 5–7 minutes until brown.

2. In a medium sauté pan over medium heat, sauté the mushrooms for 3–5 minutes.

3. Beat the eggs in a medium bowl. Add the tomatoes, beef, and mushrooms to the bowl.

4. Pour the egg mixture into a large omelet pan and cook until the omelet sets, about 5–7 minutes on medium heat.

South of the Border Scrambler

This is an easier scrambled version of Huevos Rancheros that can be made when time is short. Spice it up with jalapeños for a more authentic experience.

INGREDIENTS | SERVES 2

4 eggs (organic free-range preferred)
¼ cup salsa (see sidebar)
½ avocado, diced
¼ cup chopped fresh cilantro

Simple Salsa Recipe

Here's a simple recipe for homemade salsa: Combine 2 tomatoes, ½ jalapeño seeded, a few cilantro branches, the juice of ½ lemon, ¼ teaspoon salt, and pepper to taste. Put all ingredients in a blender, and blend until combined.

1. In a medium bowl, scramble the eggs.

2. Add the salsa, avocado, and cilantro to the egg mixture, and pour into a medium omelet pan. Cook over medium heat until set, about 5–7 minutes.

CHAPTER 10

Appetizers

Applesauce
122

Pink Applesauce
122

Cinnamon–Spiced Applesauce
123

Spiced Tropical Fruit
124

Mango Fruit Salad
125

Miguel's Guacamole
126

Spicy Guacamole
127

Tomato and Jicama Guacamole
128

Baba Ghanoush
129

Cucumber Relish
129

Avocado with Grapefruit and Sweet Onion Salsa
130

Guacamole Picado
131

Applesauce

Late-summer and fall apples are so flavorful, they don't need spices, but apples that are kept long into the winter will need some help.

INGREDIENTS | SERVES 4

8 medium apples
1 teaspoon cinnamon powder
⅛ teaspoon nutmeg powder

Healthy Snack

Spread some good-quality coconut oil on the warm, toasted rice cake. Spread a generous amount of your homemade applesauce on top of the oil, and sprinkle it all with cinnamon. Have this healthy snack with your favorite cup of tea or coffee.

1. Cut the apples into small pieces.

2. Add 1 cup of water to a saucepan, along with the apples and spices.

3. Cook on low heat for 20 minutes.

4. Remove from the heat and let cool.

Pink Applesauce

Pink applesauce owes its color to the effect of the lemon juice on the apple's red skin.

INGREDIENTS | SERVES 4

3 pounds red apples, such as McIntosh, or Macoun, cored and quartered
Juice of ½ lemon (about 2 tablespoons)

Use Applesauce as a Sweetener

Applesauce is an excellent sweetener for hot brown-rice cereal in the morning. Simply add a couple of spoonfuls of homemade applesauce to the cereal, stir to combine, and enjoy! For added texture and flavor, add some berries or sliced bananas.

1. In a medium saucepan, combine the apples and lemon juice.

2. Cook over medium heat, stirring occasionally, until the apples are soft and beginning to burst, 15–30 minutes, depending on the variety of apples.

3. Remove the skins using a food mill or your preferred method.

4. Use the applesauce immediately or store it, refrigerated, in an airtight container for up to 5 days.

Cinnamon–Spiced Applesauce

An apple a day keeps the doctor away and what better way to get that daily apple than through applesauce. Don't overdo it on a candida diet plan, however, as the preparation process can make it easier to absorb the sugars.

INGREDIENTS | SERVES 4

1½ pounds apples, cored, peeled, and cut into 1" chunks

½ cup water

Juice of ½ lemon (2 tablespoons)

Pinch coarse salt

½ tablespoon cinnamon powder

½ tablespoon nutmeg

Infuse Your Own Flavors

You may enhance the flavor of your applesauce by replacing the plain water with your favorite tea, or by boiling a stick of cinnamon in the water for 15–20 minutes or until the water turns a light brown. This trick will bring wonderful flavors to your applesauce. Try peppercorns, cardamom, or any other aromatic spice.

1. In a medium saucepan, combine the apples, water, lemon juice, and salt over a medium heat.

2. Cook, stirring and mashing the apples with the back of a wooden spoon, until the apples are soft and the water has evaporated, around 10–15 minutes.

3. Add the cinnamon and nutmeg. Combine everything together.

Spiced Tropical Fruit

This is a colorful, fun, and healthful way to create a snack that you can enjoy over 2 or 3 days.

2 ripe mangoes, sliced

2 small ripe papayas, sliced

1 ripe pineapple, sliced into strips

2 ripe bananas, sliced

3 ripe kiwis, sliced

8 ripe strawberries, sliced

1 tablespoon ground cinnamon

¼ teaspoon ground cardamom

¼ teaspoon nutmeg

¼ teaspoon allspice

1. Combine the fruit on a large platter.

2. Sprinkle the cinnamon, cardamom, nutmeg, and allspice and mix until the spices and fruits have incorporated.

Pineapple Presentation

Give this delicious tropical fruit salad a beautiful presentation by serving it inside a delectable pineapple bowl. Cut the top off the ripe pineapple, and remove the inside fruit until you end up with a bowl shape. Prepare your salad and pour it inside the pineapple bowl.

Mango Fruit Salad

Mangoes are the most popular fruit in the world and a great addition to any candida diet plan. They are rich in vitamins, antioxidants, fiber, and flavor. Outside the United States, they're known as the King of Fruits!

INGREDIENTS | SERVES 6

2 ripe mangoes
1 pineapple
1 Asian or red pear
1 pint raspberries
Juice of 1 lime
1 tablespoon freshly grated ginger

Try a Fruit Kebab

There is always a way to make your healthful dishes more appetizing. At the grocery store, buy wooden skewers or sticks, put all your fruit pieces onto the skewers, following the same pattern for every skewer.

1. Cut the fruit into bite-size pieces (except the raspberries).

2. Combine them in a medium bowl with the raspberries. In a separate small bowl, mix the juice and the ginger.

3. Add the juice mixture to the fruit, and toss gently. Serve chilled.

Miguel's Guacamole

Guacamole is an excellent appetizer and goes well with brown rice cakes, salted or unsalted.

INGREDIENTS | SERVES 6

3 ripe avocados

1 teaspoon lime juice

⅛ teaspoon salt

½ teaspoon garlic powder

½ cup chopped tomatoes

¼ cup chopped cilantro to taste

Salvadoran Guacamole

It is always a good idea to keep a few hard-boiled eggs in the refrigerator. In El Salvador, guacamole comes fortified with eggs, which makes it a healthful and complete protein appetizer. Simply mash two hard-boiled eggs into the guacamole and serve it on top of rice cakes.

1. Skin and pit the avocados. In a medium bowl, mash the fruit with a fork to your preferred consistency.

2. Blend in the lime juice, salt, and garlic powder.

3. Chop the tomatoes, and add them to the lime juice mixture.

4. Wash, dry, and chop the cilantro, and add it to the mixture. Blend the mixture and chill it.

Spicy Guacamole

Try adding turmeric, cumin, and coriander for an Indian variation of this Mexican classic.

INGREDIENTS | SERVES 4

1 small onion, chopped
2 ripe avocados
¼ teaspoon black pepper
⅛ teaspoon cayenne
Juice of 1 lemon
1 teaspoon salt
1 medium tomato, peeled, seeded, diced

1. Place the onion in a small bowl.

2. Skin and pit the avocados and add to the onion. Add the black pepper, cayenne, lemon juice, and salt. Mix well.

3. Add the tomato and stir to blend.

4. If not served immediately, cover the guacamole with plastic wrap and refrigerate it to prevent the surface from darkening.

Tomato and Jicama Guacamole

If you prefer some heat in your guacamole, the cooling effect of the avocado and tomatoes can be heated up with extra spices and jalapeños.

INGREDIENTS | SERVES 4

1 pint cherry or grape tomatoes, halved, or 2 medium tomatoes, coarsely chopped

1 medium jicama, peeled and coarsely chopped

2 avocados, coarsely chopped

¼ cup red onion, chopped

1½ tablespoons lime juice

1 teaspoon freshly grated lime rind

½ teaspoon ground cumin

⅛ teaspoon salt

⅛ teaspoon black pepper

Combine the tomatoes, jicama, avocado, red onions, lime juice and rind, and cumin in a medium bowl. Season with salt and pepper.

Jicama

If you are allergic to onion, or simply don't like it, but still want to get the crunchy texture of onion, try jicama. Also known as Mexican yam, jicama adds a crunchy, fresh taste to guacamole or pico de gallo.

Baba Ghanoush

Baba Ghanoush makes an excellent dip or spread. Use it on top of rice cakes or break the rice cakes into small pieces and dip them as you would pita bread.

INGREDIENTS | SERVES 8

4 medium eggplants
2 tablespoons fresh lemon juice
2 teaspoons chopped fresh garlic
¼ teaspoon sea salt

1. Preheat the oven to 400°F.

2. Roast the eggplants on a roasting pan for 25–30 minutes until tender and brown.

3. When cool, peel the eggplants, and process them in a food processor with the remaining ingredients.

4. Serve the dip either at room temperature or chilled.

Cucumber Relish

This recipe can be made one day ahead and stored in the refrigerator. Salt brings the moisture out of the cucumber, so if you are planning to make it early, do not salt the relish until you are ready to serve it. Use Cucumber Relish as a topping for your favorite burger or steak.

INGREDIENTS | SERVES 8

½ teaspoon cumin seeds
2 cucumbers, peeled, seeded, and cut into ¼" pieces
2 stalks of celery, washed and finely chopped
1 bunch scallions, thinly sliced
2 poblano chilies (use green bell peppers for no heat), seeds and ribs removed, finely chopped
¼ cup finely chopped fresh cilantro
3 tablespoons fresh lemon juice
¼ teaspoon coarse salt

1. Toast the cumin seeds in a small skillet over medium heat until they are lightly brown, about 3–5 minutes. Transfer the toasted seeds into a separate plate or bowl and let cool.

2. In a large bowl, combine cucumbers, celery, scallions, poblano chilies or green bell peppers, cilantro, lemon juice, and toasted cumin seeds.

3. Season with salt, and serve immediately.

Avocado with Grapefruit and Sweet Onion Salsa

Avocados are an excellent source of vitamins. There's no need to worry about getting too much fat with avocados, as their unique fats are anti-inflammatory and support the antioxidants in this superfood.

INGREDIENTS | SERVES 4

2 pink grapefruits

¼ cup finely chopped sweet onion

2 tablespoons chopped fresh cilantro

¼ teaspoon coarse salt

2 avocados, cut in half, pitted, and peeled

1. Peel the grapefruits with a paring knife. Use the knife to carefully slice between the sections and membranes of each grapefruit to remove the segments. Slice each grapefruit segment into small pieces and set aside.

2. Place the onion in a small bowl and squeeze the remaining juice from the grapefruit membranes over the onion. Let stand 20 minutes to soften.

3. Pour off the juice and discard it. Add the grapefruit segments and cilantro. Season with salt.

4. To serve, place 3–4 tablespoons on each of the avocado halves.

Guacamole Picado

This recipe comes courtesy of Priscila Satkoff, from Salpicón restaurant, Chicago, Illinois.

INGREDIENTS | MAKES 2 CUPS

1 cup diced plum tomatoes (or about 2 medium tomatoes)

¼ cup finely chopped onion

4 ounces fresh lime juice

½ cup finely chopped cilantro

1 tablespoon finely chopped serrano chilies

2 medium avocados, peeled and diced

1 tablespoon extra-virgin olive oil

Salt to taste

1. In a large bowl, mix the tomato, onion, lime juice, cilantro, and chilies.

2. Add the diced avocado and mix with the olive oil and salt to taste.

3. Cover and refrigerate for approximately 1 hour. Serve.

CHAPTER 11

Sauces and Marinades

Salsa Fresca
134

Pineapple Salsa
134

Salsa Verde
135

Pico de Gallo
136

Tomato Sauce with Basil
137

Marinara Sauce
138

Porcini Sauce
139

Hot Sauce
140

Ranchero Sauce
141

Tomato-Mint Sauce
142

Puttanesca Sauce
143

Ginger Sauce
144

Green Herb Sauce
145

Homemade Mayonnaise
146

Roasted Bell Pepper Mayonnaise
146

Hugo's Emerald Mayonnaise
147

Jalapeño Blender Mayonnaise
148

Flank Steak Marinade
149

Basil and Sage Steak Sauce
150

Salsa Fresca

Tomatoes are a rich source of antioxidants for the eyes. With more than 100 varieties of tomatoes, the flavor combinations are endless.

INGREDIENTS | SERVES 8

4 medium tomatoes, chopped

3 sprigs cilantro, chopped

½ medium onion, chopped

2 green chilies, chopped

½ lemon juice

½ teaspoon salt

1 teaspoon freshly ground pepper

Combine all the ingredients in a large bowl.

Make It a Dipping Salsa

After week 13, turn this recipe into a dipping sauce for chips or a sauce for scrambled eggs. Just blend all the ingredients in a blender.

Pineapple Salsa

This is a Hawaiian variation of the Mexican classic. Adding pineapple enhances the nutritional benefits of the tomatoes and spices and adds sweetness.

INGREDIENTS | SERVES 8

3 cups peeled and diced pineapple

1 small red onion, chopped

1 small bell pepper of any color, seeds and ribs removed, diced

2 poblano chilies or jalapeños for more heat, seeds and ribs removed, finely chopped

½ cup rinsed, finely chopped fresh cilantro

2 tablespoons finely chopped fresh mint, approximately

½ teaspoon coarse salt

½ teaspoon freshly ground pepper

1. Combine all ingredients in a large bowl. Let the mixture stand at least 30 minutes to allow the flavors to develop.

2. Serve or store covered in plastic wrap in the refrigerator for up to 1 day.

Salsa Verde

The green cousin of Salsa Fresca, Salsa Verde is typically made with tomatillos instead of tomatoes and tends to have a texture that is less chunky.

INGREDIENTS | SERVES 4

1 pound tomatillos, cooked, peeled, and chopped

½ medium onion, chopped

3 sprigs cilantro, chopped

½ teaspoon coarse salt

½ teaspoon freshly ground pepper

Combine all the ingredients in a medium bowl and serve or store in the fridge for up to 5 days.

Italian Style

Italy has its own take on Salsa Verde. Typical ingredients of the Italian version include parsley, basil, anchovies, capers, olive oil, and Dijon mustard. It is delicious with seared and roasted meats.

Pico de Gallo

Pico de Gallo is a Mexican classic. Add some fresh corn, avocado, or spices like cinnamon, cumin, and parsley for slight variations in the textures and flavors.

INGREDIENTS | SERVES 8

1 medium white onion, diced
4 large tomatoes, chopped
1 large jalapeño, seeded and minced
¼ cup freshly squeezed lime juice
½ cup finely chopped cilantro
½ teaspoon coarse salt
½ teaspoon freshly ground pepper

1. Combine the ingredients in a bowl and allow to marinate for 30 minutes.

2. Serve or store in the refrigerator.

Tropical Variation

You can give this recipe a tropical twist by replacing the tomatoes with fresh sweet mango. Mango Pico de Gallo is becoming very popular in Mexican-American cuisine. Try it with your next grilled protein.

Tomato Sauce with Basil

A classic Italian sauce, this works well with most meats and veggies. You can also use it over spaghetti squash or heat it up with chilies.

INGREDIENTS | SERVES 6

12 large vine-ripened tomatoes (about 6½ cups)
2 tablespoons olive oil
1 tablespoon chopped fresh garlic
½ cup vegetable stock
¼ cup chopped fresh basil
⅛ teaspoon sea salt
¼ teaspoon ground pepper

Canned Salsa

Did you know that most canned or jarred salsas sold at grocery stores are cooked to a temperature of 175°F to increase their shelf life? Make your salsa fresh and refrigerate it immediately. Canned products are not recommended during the first nine weeks of the candida diet.

1. Boil a large pot of water. Remove the tomato cores and place the tomatoes in boiling water for 2 minutes. Remove the tomatoes and place them in cold water. When they are cool enough to handle, peel the tomatoes and squeeze them gently to remove the seeds. Discard the seeds and cut the tomatoes into large dice.

2. Lightly coat a large sauté pan with the olive oil and place over low heat. Add the garlic and cook, stirring, for 1 minute.

3. Add the chopped tomatoes and vegetable stock.

4. Cover and cook gently over low heat for 20 minutes. Stir in the fresh basil and season with salt and pepper.

Marinara Sauce

An excellent way to liven up a dish of spaghetti squash or pour some Marinara Sauce over ground beef and veggies!

INGREDIENTS | MAKES 3 CUPS

2 tablespoons olive oil

1 large onion, chopped

1½ tablespoons finely chopped fresh garlic

1½ teaspoons dried basil

1 teaspoon dried oregano

4 cups chopped tomatoes, puréed

1. Add the olive oil to a large saucepan, and set on low heat. Add the onions and cook, stirring often, until they begin to soften, about 2 minutes.

2. Add the garlic, basil, and oregano, and stir for 15 seconds.

3. Stir in the tomatoes. Cover and cook for 25 minutes, stirring often. Serve.

Candida-Friendly Pasta

This sauce makes an excellent topping for spaghetti squash. Cook the sauce with some ground beef seasoned with salt, pepper, and dried herbs. When the beef is fully cooked, add the Marinara Sauce, and serve it with spaghetti squash or steamed vegetables.

Porcini Sauce

Porcini mushrooms have a hearty flavor; the dried mushrooms are typically more flavorful than the fresh. Try using the fresh mushrooms if you desire a more subtle flavor.

INGREDIENTS | SERVES 6

2 ounces dried porcini mushrooms

½ cup warm water

5 cloves garlic, peeled and chopped

1 tablespoon olive oil

1 tablespoon finely chopped fresh thyme

1 tablespoon finely chopped fresh rosemary

1 cup tomato sauce

½ teaspoon coarse salt

½ teaspoon freshly ground pepper

Mushrooms and Candida

Some people are concerned about mushrooms feeding the candida, but it has not been determined that mushrooms create candida fungus in the human body. Eat from the Yes Foods in moderation, and see what works for you. If you react to a certain food, don't eat it.

1. Soften the dried porcini in warm water for 30 minutes.

2. Add the garlic cloves to a medium sauté pan and gently sauté in the olive oil over medium heat for 2–3 minutes.

3. Add the thyme, rosemary, tomato sauce, salt, and pepper.

4. Strain the mushroom water through a cheesecloth, and then add it to the tomato mixture.

5. Chop and add the mushrooms.

6. Simmer the sauce over medium-low heat until thick and savory, about 20 minutes. Serve.

Hot Sauce

This is a hotter version of Salsa Fresca. If you're a hot pepper aficionado, you'll have fun seeing how hot you can make your homemade sauce.

INGREDIENTS | MAKES 4 CUPS

5 large vine-ripened tomatoes
1 serrano chili
1 tablespoon chopped fresh parsley
¼ teaspoon chopped fresh garlic
⅛ teaspoon sea salt

Need More Heat?

You may modify this recipe based on your level of heat preference. If you want extreme heat, go with a habañero pepper. The habañero is one of the spiciest chilies out there. Try a jalapeño or other varieties. Experiment with the chilies and see which you prefer.

1. Preheat the oven to 350°F.

2. Set the tomatoes and pepper in a baking dish. Roast them in the oven until the skins blister, about 25 minutes. Let cool, and then peel the pepper.

3. Purée the tomatoes (with skin on) and pepper in a food processor.

4. Stir in the parsley, garlic, and salt. Serve.

Ranchero Sauce

Sauces are a great way to add more spices to any meal. Don't be afraid to take advantage of their many healing properties.

INGREDIENTS | SERVES 8

4 medium tomatoes, chopped
1 medium onion, chopped
2 garlic cloves, chopped
¼ jalapeño, stemmed and chopped
¼ teaspoon salt
¼ teaspoon chili powder
1½ teaspoons dried oregano
½ cup water

1. Add the tomatoes, onions, garlic, and jalapeño to a medium frying pan.

2. Add the salt, chili powder, oregano, and water.

3. Cook over medium heat until the tomatoes and onions are soft, about 6 minutes.

4. Purée half of mixture in a blender. Transfer to a bowl and stir in the remaining sauce that was not puréed. Serve.

Tomato-Mint Sauce

This is a great sauce, hot or cold. Serving this sauce hot is delicious on those colder days, while serving it cold is very refreshing during the summer months.

INGREDIENTS | SERVES 6

½ medium yellow onion, chopped

2 cloves garlic, crushed

2 teaspoons dried mint, or ½ cup fresh mint

2–3 cups fresh spinach (optional)

3 tablespoons olive oil

1½ cups diced fresh tomatoes

¼ teaspoon salt, or to taste

¼ teaspoon pepper, or to taste

1. In a medium sauté pan, sauté the onion, garlic, mint, and spinach, if used, in olive oil for 5 minutes over medium heat.

2. Add the tomatoes to the mix and cook for 15 minutes.

3. Season with the salt and pepper and serve.

Tomato-Mint Soup

To make this soup, place all the cooked ingredients in a blender and process until the texture is like a purée. Eat this wonderful soup (or sauce) as a side dish or appetizer. Try it on top of baked chicken or sautéed vegetables.

Puttanesca Sauce

This flavorful sauce has an abundance of healing spices. Experiment with the flavor even more by adding a cup of green or kalamata olives and a quarter cup of capers.

INGREDIENTS | SERVES 6

⅓ cup olive oil

1 tablespoon minced garlic

4 cups fresh chopped plum tomatoes, drained

1 tablespoon minced fresh oregano

½ teaspoon red pepper flakes

2 ounces minced anchovies

¼ teaspoon salt, or to taste

¼ teaspoon pepper, or to taste

1 pound cooked brown rice

2 tablespoons minced fresh parsley

2 tablespoons minced fresh basil

Alternative to Pasta

Short- or long-grain brown rice makes an excellent and healthful alternative to pasta. Make any sauce that you would normally put on pasta and pour it over brown rice. Note: Brown rice pasta is not allowed on the plan until week 13.

1. In a large saucepan, add the olive oil and minced garlic. Sauté briefly over medium heat for 2 minutes.

2. Add the plum tomatoes, fresh oregano, and red pepper flakes. Cover the pan and simmer the sauce for 10 minutes.

3. Uncover and simmer for another 10 minutes, stirring occasionally.

4. To the reduced sauce, add the anchovies, and season with the salt and pepper.

5. Simmer 5 minutes longer to heat through and blend the flavors.

6. In a large bowl, add the sauce to the rice, and sprinkle with the parsley and basil.

Ginger Sauce

Ginger is a great spice for adding warmth to any dish, and it aids digestion.

INGREDIENTS | SERVES 4

1 (½"-thick) gingerroot, peeled, minced
½ cup Homemade Mayonnaise (see recipe later in this chapter)
2 teaspoons chopped cilantro leaves
2 teaspoons lime juice
¼ teaspoon hot chili oil

1. Combine all the ingredients in a small bowl.

2. Refrigerate until ready to serve.

Dipping Sauce

This is an excellent dipping sauce for steamed shrimp, baked salmon, or any other seafood dish. You may also use it with chicken. This recipe calls for Homemade Mayonnaise; however, after week 9, you may use jarred (store-bought) mayonnaise.

Green Herb Sauce

This is a tasty way to enjoy the healing properties of herbs and spices.

INGREDIENTS | SERVES 4

2 lemons
5 garlic cloves, finely chopped
1 cup chopped fresh cilantro
1 cup chopped fresh basil
½ cup chopped fresh parsley
1 cup olive oil
1 teaspoon salt
½ teaspoon pepper

1. In a small bowl, grate the zest from both lemons. Halve and squeeze juice into bowl.

2. Add the chopped garlic to the lemon juice and zest.

3. Stir in the chopped cilantro, basil, and parsley. Add the olive oil, stirring until blended.

4. Add the salt and pepper. Serve at room temperature.

Use It as a Marinade

This sauce makes a delicious marinade for any meat. To prepare, make the sauce, choose your meat, place it into a large zippered bag, pour the marinade into the bag, seal and place in the refrigerator overnight. Grill it, bake it, or pan-fry it.

Homemade Mayonnaise

Store-bought mayonnaise won't work well on a candida diet plan due to the vinegar and sugars they often contain, but homemade varieties can taste even better and be more nutritious.

INGREDIENTS | MAKES 2 CUPS

2 egg yolks
½ teaspoon salt
1 teaspoon dry mustard
3 tablespoons lemon juice
1¼ cups olive oil

1. Put all ingredients, except the oil, in the food processor. Process for a few seconds.

2. Turn off the machine and scrape down the sides.

3. With the machine running, add the oil in a thin stream. Blend until thick.

Roasted Bell Pepper Mayonnaise

Roasted peppers are great right from the oven, or they can be stored in olive oil in the refrigerator for up to 2 weeks. Add roasted peppers to salads, main dishes, or eggs, or eat them by themselves.

INGREDIENTS | MAKES 3 CUPS

4 bell peppers
2 cups Homemade Mayonnaise (see recipe earlier in this chapter)

1. Preheat the oven to 500°F.

2. Halve the peppers and remove the seeds and ribs. Place the cut-side down on a baking sheet and roast until charred, about 15 minutes. Cool, peel, and slice.

3. Put the roasted peppers and Homemade Mayonnaise into a blender. Blend until combined and serve.

Hugo's Emerald Mayonnaise

Inspired by Italy's rolling green hills, this recipe is filled with vital nutrients and antioxidants that can turn any dish into an infusion of health.

INGREDIENTS | MAKES 1 CUP

2 eggs, at room temperature

2 tablespoons fresh lemon juice

½ teaspoon salt

¼ cup oil

¼ cup snipped chives

4 parsley sprigs

½ teaspoon dried tarragon

½ teaspoon dried thyme

1 scallion, chopped

½ cup spinach, watercress, or sorrel

½ teaspoon mustard powder

1. Combine the eggs, lemon juice, and salt in a blender, and blend at high speed for 1 minute.

2. Slowly add the oil in a thin stream until the ingredients are mixed and thicken. Remove the mayonnaise from the blender and pour it into a medium bowl.

3. Process the remaining ingredients in the blender. Move the ingredients to a large bowl, add the mayonnaise, and whisk the ingredients.

4. Refrigerate in a glass jar and use as you would any other mayonnaise.

Jalapeño Blender Mayonnaise

Add a little spice to your diet with this hot condiment. A little goes a long way with this one.

INGREDIENTS | MAKES 1 CUP

2 egg yolks, at room temperature

½ teaspoon sea salt

1 teaspoon dry mustard

3 tablespoons lemon juice

¼ cup olive oil

½ slice of raw jalapeño cut lengthwise, with veins and seeds

Variations

Experiment with mayonnaise. Try adding one roasted bell pepper into your mixture. Another variation is garlic mayo. Simply add 2 minced garlic cloves to the rest of your ingredients, simple and delicious.

1. Put all ingredients, except the oil, into the food processor or blender.

2. Mix for a few seconds until well blended.

3. Turn off the blender and scrap the sides with a spatula.

4. With the blender or processor running, add the oil in a thin stream. Blend until thick. Refrigerate between uses.

5. Add the jalapeño, and blend for 30 seconds until the mayo looks slightly green.

Flank Steak Marinade

Bragg Liquid Aminos is a healthful, non-GMO substitute for soy sauces. It can be used with meats, veggies, eggs, soups, and salad dressings.

INGREDIENTS | MAKES 1 CUP

1½ teaspoons salt

1 tablespoon minced onion

½ teaspoon dry mustard

½ teaspoon rosemary

¼ teaspoon powdered ginger

¼ cup lemon juice

½ cup olive oil

1 clove garlic, minced

¼ cup Bragg Liquid Aminos

1 teaspoon ground black pepper

1. Place all ingredients in blender and blend until smooth.

2. Let marinade set overnight in the fridge before adding meat.

Tip

Flank steak does well when left to marinate overnight. Some people like to add an acidic agent such as lemon to break down the tissue before cooking. Once cooked, allow the flank steak to sit for a few minutes to let the juices settle. Always cut against the grain.

Basil and Sage Steak Sauce

This is an easy recipe that can be made just prior to grilling or cooking your steak.

INGREDIENTS | SERVES 2

4 tablespoons olive oil
¼ cup packed fresh sage leaves
¼ cup packed fresh basil leaves

Cooking Tip

When cooking steak, make sure that the pan or grill is very hot. Do not press on the steak; this will squeeze out the juices and make the steak dry. Flip the steak only once. After the steak is cooked, let it rest for a few minutes before cutting it to allow the juices to distribute inside.

1. Combine the oil, sage, and basil in small saucepan.

2. Cook over medium heat about 10 minutes.

3. Strain the sage and basil leaves. Refrigerate and store up to 3 days.

CHAPTER 12

Salads

Spiced Crab and Avocado Salad
152

Tuna and Avocado Spread
153

Egg Salad
153

Maryellen's Tuna Salad
154

Fresh Tuna with Watercress Salad
155

Tuna Salad with Beefsteak Tomatoes
156

Spiced Crab and Avocado Salad

This spicier version of a New England classic is delicious as a snack or combined with a dinner.

INGREDIENTS | SERVES 4

3 tablespoons Homemade Mayonnaise
 (see recipe in Chapter 11)

2 tablespoons lime juice

1 teaspoon cumin

½ teaspoon paprika

1 pound crabmeat, cooked

2 celery stalks, sliced

½ teaspoon salt

½ teaspoon pepper

1 avocado, pitted, peeled, and cubed

2 bunches watercress, stems removed

1. Mix the mayonnaise, lime juice, cumin, and paprika in a large bowl.

2. Add the crabmeat and celery. Season with salt and pepper. Add the avocado, being careful not to crush the cubes.

3. Place the watercress on the plates, top with the crab-avocado mixture, and serve.

Open-Face Sandwich

Use this delicious crab and avocado salad as a topping for an open-face sandwich. Toast a plain rice cake for 2 minutes, spread the salad on top of the rice cake, and sprinkle with a little cayenne pepper for a kick.

Tuna and Avocado Spread

You can spice up this simple recipe with chipotle peppers, garlic powder, dill, cilantro, basil, lemon, or turmeric.

INGREDIENTS | SERVES 2

1 (5-ounce can) chunk light tuna in water

1 ripe avocado

½ teaspoon garlic powder

⅛ teaspoon cayenne pepper

½ teaspoon dried basil

In a small bowl, combine the tuna, the avocado, and the spices. Mash to a desired consistency with a fork and serve.

Egg Salad

Eggs are a superfood any time of day. Packed with protein, antioxidants, and beneficial fats, eggs help make any meal or snack healthful. Serve this recipe on top of spinach or salad greens.

INGREDIENTS | SERVES 4

6 hard-boiled, organic, free-range eggs, peeled and chopped

1 stalk celery, chopped

3 medium green onions, chopped

½ green or red pepper, minced

¼ cup Homemade Mayonnaise (see recipe in Chapter 11)

⅛ teaspoon each of marjoram, sweet basil, cayenne, garlic powder, pepper, oregano, dill weed

Chili powder to taste (optional)

In a medium bowl, combine the hard-boiled eggs, celery, onions, and peppers. Add the mayonnaise and mix again. Add the spices to taste.

Maryellen's Tuna Salad

White albacore tuna packed in water can be a heart-healthy choice of omega-3 fatty acids for salads and meals.

INGREDIENTS | SERVES 2

1 (5-ounce) can white albacore tuna packed in water

¼ cup chopped green olives

2 medium green onions, diced

½ teaspoon mustard powder

2 tablespoons chopped red pepper

¼ teaspoon salt

½ teaspoon pepper

1 hard-boiled, organic, free-range egg, chopped

2 cups mixed greens

In a medium bowl, mix all the ingredients until blended. Serve over greens.

Fresh Tuna with Watercress Salad

Watercress is a good source of folates, vitamins, antioxidants, and minerals that can help increase the heart-healthy benefits of tuna.

INGREDIENTS | SERVES 5

5 tablespoons Bragg Liquid Aminos

¼ cup fresh cilantro leaves (packed)

2 tablespoons Homemade Mayonnaise (see recipe in Chapter 11)

1 tablespoon sesame oil

2 teaspoons lime juice

1 (1") piece peeled fresh ginger, chopped

¼ teaspoon cayenne pepper

2 (6-ounce) fillets tuna

2 bunches watercress, stems trimmed

1 bunch radishes, trimmed, sliced

1 tablespoon sesame seeds

1. Blend the Bragg Liquid Aminos, cilantro, mayonnaise, sesame oil, lime juice, ginger, and cayenne pepper in blender until smooth.

2. Pour ⅓ cup of the sauce into a glass pie plate, add the fish, and turn to coat, 15 minutes per side.

3. Reserve the remaining sauce for later use.

4. Drain the marinade from the tuna into a heavy medium skillet. Cook the liquid on high until it starts to boil.

5. Add the tuna and cook about 3 minutes per side for medium-rare.

6. Combine the watercress and radishes in a bowl and arrange the fish slices on top.

7. Sprinkle with the sesame seeds and reserved marinade.

Tuna Salad with Beefsteak Tomatoes

Beefsteak tomatoes generally come by the pound. Thick and juicy like steaks, beefsteak tomatoes are a great addition to tuna salads.

INGREDIENTS | SERVES 4

2 (5-ounce) cans white albacore tuna packed in water

2 tablespoons chicken broth

1 tablespoon fresh lemon juice

¼ cup Homemade Mayonnaise (see recipe in Chapter 11)

½ teaspoon salt, divided

½ teaspoon pepper, divided

2 large ripe tomatoes, sliced ¼" thick

1. Mix the tuna, chicken broth, and lemon juice in a food processor. Remove to a medium bowl and fold in the mayonnaise.

2. Season with ¼ teaspoon salt and ¼ teaspoon pepper. Cover and chill at least 1 hour.

3. Slice the tomatoes, and sprinkle with the remaining salt and pepper.

4. Serve a scoop of the tuna mixture on top of each tomato.

CHAPTER 13

Lunch

Lettuce and Beef
158

Tuna Salad Roll-Up
159

Chunky Chicken Salad
160

Niçoise Salad
161

Pineapple, Red Pepper, and Brown Rice Salad
162

South American Chili
163

Lettuce and Beef

In this take on the American burger classic, lettuce leaves take the place of bread. This version is delicious any time of day.

INGREDIENTS | SERVES 4

1 pound ground beef

¼ teaspoon salt

¼ teaspoon black pepper

5 tablespoons Bragg Liquid Aminos

2 teaspoons chopped parsley

2 teaspoons chopped dill

2 teaspoons chopped tarragon

¼ cup Homemade Mayonnaise (see recipe in Chapter 11), plus more for topping (optional)

1 head butter lettuce

1 large tomato, sliced

1 avocado, sliced

1 slice red onion

1. Place the beef in a bowl and add salt, pepper, and 3 tablespoons of Bragg Liquid Aminos. Knead the ingredients to combine.

2. Shape the beef into 4 medium-size patties.

3. Cook them on the grill or in a skillet over medium-high heat (3 minutes for medium-rare on the grill, 3½ minutes for medium-rare in a pan).

4. Mix the parsley, dill, tarragon, and 2 tablespoons Bragg Liquid Aminos in a small bowl. Add the mayonnaise and mix again. Put aside.

5. Wash the lettuce and remove 8 leaves. Place one leaf on each plate.

6. Add 1 burger patty to each lettuce leaf, and layer the tomato, avocado, and onion slices on top.

7. Add the mayonnaise mixture and serve.

Tuna Salad Roll-Up

This is a tasty recipe that has some crunch. Roll-ups are a fun alternative to a sandwich and are easy to assemble and take with you.

INGREDIENTS | SERVES 3

1 (ounce) can white albacore tuna packed in water

2 tablespoons Homemade Mayonnaise (see recipe in Chapter 11)

1 medium apple, diced

½ medium red onion, finely diced

2 sticks chopped celery

1 hard-boiled, organic, free-range egg, diced

3 lettuce leaves

1. In a medium bowl, thoroughly mix all the ingredients, except the lettuce.

2. Place a scoop of tuna salad on each lettuce leaf, roll up, and serve.

Tips for Making Good Burgers

Burgers need some fat in order to be juicy. Using lean beef can result in a dry burger. The ideal meat will be freshly ground chuck with 10–18 percent fat content. In addition to using good meat, don't flip your burgers too often, as this will also make them drier. Only flip the burgers once.

Chunky Chicken Salad

This is delicious when served in lettuce leaf or collards greens.

INGREDIENTS | SERVES 4

4 skinless and boneless chicken breasts

2 cups chicken stock

1 red pepper, cut into ¼" pieces

1 yellow pepper, cut into ¼" pieces

1 orange pepper, cut into ¼" pieces

½ cup Homemade Mayonnaise (see recipe in Chapter 11)

1 tablespoon fresh tarragon, coarsely chopped

1 tablespoon fresh chives

1. In a large saucepan, gently poach the chicken breasts in stock over medium heat for about 20 minutes, being careful not to overcook.

2. Remove the chicken from the stock, let cool, and then cut into chunks.

3. In a large bowl, toss the peppers and chicken in mayonnaise.

4. Add the tarragon and toss again. Top with chives.

Chicken Safety

When cooking with chicken, you must be very careful not to cross contaminate surfaces, so make sure to have one designated cutting board for your chicken, and a separate one for your vegetables. Unlike beef, chicken must be cooked all the way through to prevent any food poisoning.

Niçoise Salad

This Mediterranean delight is packed with vitamins that will keep you going all day. This simple recipe allows for a lot of experimentation with spices.

INGREDIENTS | SERVES 5

1 large head butter lettuce greens

3 (5-ounce) cans white albacore tuna packed in water

10 small roasted potatoes

½ pound green beans

10 hard-boiled eggs

4 medium tomatoes

½ cup olives niçoise

½ cup olive oil

½ cup lemon juice

1. Place the lettuce leaves on a plate as a bed. Put the tuna in the center of the plate.

2. Boil the potatoes in a stockpot for 6 minutes over medium-high heat. Remove the potatoes and set aside.

3. Boil the green beans in the stockpot over medium heat for 3 minutes to tenderize them. Remove the beans and set aside.

4. Slice the eggs, potatoes, and tomatoes. Arrange each along the perimeter of the plate.

5. Chop the green beans into ½-inch pieces. Add to the arrangement along with the olives.

6. Sprinkle with the olive oil and lemon juice to taste. Serve.

Pineapple, Red Pepper, and Brown Rice Salad

This is a sweet and spicy version of brown rice that is sure to please your taste buds.

INGREDIENTS | SERVES 6

4 cups cooked brown rice

1 cup diced fresh pineapple

1 tablespoon lemon or lime juice, plus 1 teaspoon

½ teaspoon hot chili oil

½ cup diced red bell pepper

½ cup green onions with some tops

1 teaspoon sesame oil

½ teaspoon salt

1 tablespoon olive oil, plus 1 teaspoon

1. Put the cooked brown rice in a large bowl; stir in the pineapple.

2. Add lemon or lime juice, chili oil, bell pepper, green onions, sesame oil, salt, and olive oil.

3. Toss to mix.

South American Chili

This makes a great hot lunch meal on cold winter days. Make a large batch, even if there are only one or two people who'll eat it. Store the extra in the fridge and take it with you, add rice cakes for some crunch at the last minute, or spread it over spaghetti squash.

INGREDIENTS | SERVES 8–10

2 tablespoons olive oil

2 cups onions

2 cups chopped red bell peppers

4 large garlic cloves, minced

2 pounds ground beef

1 tablespoon cumin

1 teaspoon cayenne pepper, plus more to taste

1¼–1½ ounces beef broth

1 cup peas

1 cup freshly diced tomatoes

½ tablespoon salt

1. Heat the oil in a large pot over medium-high. Add the onions, bell peppers, and garlic, and sauté for 5 minutes.

2. Add the ground beef, cumin, and cayenne pepper. Sauté until the ground beef is brown, breaking up the beef with the back of a fork, about 8 minutes.

3. Add the beef broth, peas, and tomatoes. Simmer until the chili is thick, stirring occasionally, about 20 minutes.

4. Season with cayenne pepper and salt to taste.

CHAPTER 14

Soups and Stews

Chicken Stock
166

Vegetable Stock
167

Guacamole Soup
168

Avocado-Zucchini Soup
169

Gazpacho
170

Potato-Leek Soup
171

Chicken Soup with Asparagus
172

Lime-Cilantro Soup
173

Beet Soup
174

Vegetable Chowder
175

Harvest Vegetable Stew
176

Slow-Cooker Mediterranean Stew
177

Nikki's Stew
178

Corn Soup
179

Chicken Stock

Stocks are a healthful choice to use in your dishes. Slow-cooking on low heat helps extract the most nutrients out of all foods and can turn an ordinary meal into a powerhouse of healing.

INGREDIENTS | MAKES 15 CUPS

6 pounds chicken bones, cut up (substitute chicken wings if bones or carcasses are unavailable)

4 quarts cold water

1 large onion, chopped

1 small carrot, coarsely chopped

1 small stalk celery, chopped

Beef Stock

If you want to make a beef stock, replace the chicken bones with beef bones. Adding bone marrow will make your recipe richer. For more taste, add your favorite herbs. For the chicken stock, add poultry herbs such as sage, rosemary, and thyme. Put all the herbs in a cheesecloth pouch for easy removal.

1. In a very large pot, combine the chicken bones and water. The water should cover the bones by about 2 inches.

2. Bring to a boil over medium heat. Skim off the foam that rises to the surface. Add the remaining ingredients. Reduce the heat to low, and simmer, uncovered about 6 hours.

3. Strain the stock through a sieve into a large bowl. Cool completely, cover, and refrigerate. Skim off and discard the fat that accumulates on the surface.

Vegetable Stock

Adding cold water when cooking stocks increases the flavor. Cut the vegetables into small pieces first to get the most flavor out of each piece. This stock will keep for up to 1 week in the refrigerator or for 1 month in the freezer.

INGREDIENTS | MAKES 7 CUPS

4 medium carrots, peeled and cut into chunks

2 stalks celery, tough strings peeled, stalks cut into chunks

2 medium onions, roughly chopped

1 leek, halved lengthwise and washed thoroughly

8 cups fresh water

1. In a large pot, combine all the ingredients and bring to a boil. Reduce heat to low and cook for 25 minutes.

2. Strain the stock and reserve it for soups and sauces.

Guacamole Soup

This cold blender soup can be made in 10 minutes up to 8 hours before you serve it. Guacamole Soup is a delicious first course for any summer meal.

INGREDIENTS | SERVES 4

½ cup cilantro leaves

2 green onions, cut into 1" pieces

1 jalapeño, seeded and coarsely chopped

2 cups chicken broth

½ cup puréed tomatoes

¼ cup lemon juice

2 small avocados, peeled, pitted, and coarsely chopped

½ teaspoon salt

1. In a food processor, pulse the cilantro, green onions, and jalapeño until finely chopped, scraping down the sides of the bowl as necessary.

2. Add the chicken broth, tomatoes, lemon juice, and avocados. Process until smooth. Add salt. Refrigerate 1 hour for flavors to blend.

Avocado-Zucchini Soup

Choose smaller zucchini for better flavor. If you're fortunate enough to find the edible flowers, add them as well.

INGREDIENTS | SERVES 4

2 tablespoons olive oil

4 medium green onions, chopped, divided

1 teaspoon grated fresh ginger

1 garlic clove, chopped

4 cups vegetable broth

1 cup water

2 medium zucchini, thinly sliced

½ teaspoon salt

¼ teaspoon pepper

1 medium avocado, seeded, peeled, and chopped

1 tablespoon lemon juice

1 tablespoon chopped bell pepper

1. Heat the olive oil in a medium-to-large saucepan over medium heat. Add 4 green onions and cook for 2–3 minutes. Add the ginger and garlic; cook, stirring, for 1 minute.

2. Add the vegetable broth, water, zucchini, salt, and pepper. Stir to mix the ingredients, cover, and cook until the zucchini are cooked and soft, approximately 10 minutes. Let cool for 5 minutes. Stir in the avocado.

3. Purée the soup in batches in a food processor or blender. (If you have a hand blender, there's no need to let the mixture cool. If putting in a processor, allow to cool a bit first.) Return the soup to the saucepan to heat through. Stir in the lemon juice. Garnish with the red pepper and remaining green onions.

Gazpacho

The Spanish have known for centuries that this soup, served cold, is a delicious, healthful way to cool off during the summer.

INGREDIENTS | SERVES 6

2 pounds (6 large) ripe tomatoes, chopped

1 pound (2 medium) cucumbers, peeled and chopped, plus diced for garnish

½ pound (3 medium) green peppers, seeded and chopped, plus diced for garnish

¼ pound (1 small) sweet onion, peeled and chopped

1 large clove garlic, peeled and chopped

¼ cup olive oil

2 tablespoons lime juice

2 teaspoons salt

Blending Soup

If you are using a food processor, this proportion of vegetables will make a thick, slightly crunchy soup. If you want the soup a bit thinner, add another large tomato. If you are using a blender, put the tomatoes in first, with a bit of oil and lime juice to provide the necessary liquid. Set aside several pieces of cucumber and pepper to add, diced, as a garnish when you serve the soup.

1. Purée all the ingredients in a food processor or blender in batches, leaving a little liquid in the container to start each batch. Remove to a large bowl or container.

2. Serve the gazpacho cold.

Potato-Leek Soup

Choose tender leeks and firm potatoes for the best results.

INGREDIENTS | MAKES 4 QUARTS

2 tablespoons extra-virgin olive oil

3 leeks, washed and halved

1 large onion, chopped

4 large potatoes, peeled and cut into large chunks

3 quarts Vegetable Stock (see recipe in this chapter)

⅛ teaspoon sea salt

¼ teaspoon fresh ground black pepper

2 tablespoons snipped fresh chives

1. Coat a large soup pot with the olive oil and heat over a low setting.

2. Add the leeks and onions, and cook, covered, for 10 minutes.

3. Add the potatoes and stock. Bring to boil; then reduce heat to medium-low. Simmer until the potatoes are soft, about 20 minutes.

4. Purée soup in a blender or with a hand blender. Season with salt and pepper, and garnish with chives.

Chicken Soup with Asparagus

The curative powers of chicken soup and asparagus join to make a warm and tasty powerhouse soup. Asparagus has high levels of folates that can help keep the mind sharp, so this soup is a smart choice for everyone.

INGREDIENTS | SERVES 6

7 cups Chicken Stock (see recipe in this chapter)

2 chicken breast halves (1 pound)

¾ pound asparagus spears, cut into 1½" pieces

4 cups lightly packed, thinly sliced Swiss chard leaves

4 plum tomatoes, seeded and chopped

½ teaspoon coarse salt

½ teaspoon black pepper

Add Some Variety

Use your favorite vegetables for this recipe. Try replacing the chard with spinach, kale, or collard greens. There is no way to go wrong. Adding some cubed zucchini toward the end of the cooking process gives the soup a little more texture.

1. In a 4-quart Dutch oven, combine the chicken stock and chicken. Bring to a boil, and then reduce the heat to low. Simmer, covered, for 20 minutes or until the chicken is no longer pink.

2. Remove the chicken from the broth; cool slightly. Discard the skin and bones. Shred the chicken into bite-size pieces.

3. Add the asparagus to the broth. Cook for 3 minutes.

4. Stir in the Swiss chard, tomatoes, and shredded cooked chicken. Heat through.

5. Add salt and pepper.

Lime-Cilantro Soup

Lime soup is a favorite dish from Mexico's Yucatán peninsula. The combination of lime and cilantro gives this dish plenty of zest!

INGREDIENTS | SERVES 4

2 tablespoons extra-virgin olive oil

2 garlic cloves, minced

1 medium onion, chopped

1 tablespoon chili powder

2 skinless boneless chicken breast halves

5 cups chicken broth

1 cup frozen corn kernels

2 medium tomatoes, chopped

½ bunch fresh cilantro sprigs, tied together with string

¼ cup chopped cilantro

¼ cup lime juice

½ teaspoon coarse salt

½ teaspoon black pepper

1. In large saucepan, add the oil, garlic, and onion, and cook over medium heat for 3 minutes.

2. Add the chili powder and chicken, stirring for 3 minutes.

3. Add the chicken broth, corn, tomatoes, and cilantro sprigs. Bring the soup to a boil. Reduce heat to low and simmer until chicken is cooked through, about 10 minutes.

4. Discard the cilantro sprigs.

5. Add the chopped cilantro, lime juice, salt, and pepper.

Try It with Beef

This delicious sour soup is just as good with beef. If you use stew meat, it requires at least 1 hour of cooking to become tender.

Beet Soup

Beets are a good way to cleanse and heal the body. Their colorful appearance comes from high levels of antioxidants and phytochemicals. Enjoy this soup year-round.

INGREDIENTS | SERVES 8

1 tablespoon olive oil

1 medium onion, chopped

3 cloves garlic, crushed

1 tablespoon fresh grated ginger (optional)

2 large carrots, peeled and chopped

2 stalks celery, chopped

3 medium beets, peeled and chopped

2 large potatoes, diced or cubed

4 cups salt-free chicken or vegetable broth

1 tablespoon Bragg Liquid Aminos

¼ teaspoon pepper

Give It Some Color

Combine or replace the red beets with golden beets, for a change of color. Beets are excellent for blood circulation and detoxification.

1. In a large pot, heat the olive oil over medium; then add onions and garlic (and ginger, if you are using it). Sauté until lightly browned, about 6–8 minutes.

2. Add the carrots and celery, and let the mixture cook for 5 minutes.

3. Add the beets and potatoes, and cook for 5 more minutes.

4. Add the broth, and bring to a simmer.

5. Add the Bragg Liquid Aminos and pepper to taste, and simmer for 30 minutes.

Vegetable Chowder

If you make this soup the night before you need it, add the spinach and basil when you reheat it to preserve their freshness.

INGREDIENTS | SERVES 4–6

4 stalks celery, chopped

4 medium carrots, chopped

2 tablespoons olive oil

2 zucchini, chopped

2 cups sliced mushrooms

2 bay leaves

1 tablespoon paprika

1½ teaspoons chopped basil

1 teaspoon thyme

1½ teaspoons ground ginger

1⅛ teaspoons cayenne pepper

6 cups Vegetable Stock or Chicken Stock (see recipes in this chapter)

½ teaspoon coarse salt

½ teaspoon black pepper

2 cups puréed tomatoes

1 (10-ounce) bag spinach, chopped

1. In a medium sauté pan, sauté the celery and carrots in olive oil for 10 minutes. Add the zucchini, mushrooms, bay leaves, paprika, basil, thyme, ginger, and cayenne.

2. Sauté on medium heat for 2–6 minutes, stirring to ensure the vegetables are not sticking. If they stick, turn the heat down.

3. Add stock, salt, pepper, tomatoes, and spinach. Simmer for 5 minutes.

Harvest Vegetable Stew

Harvest time is when farmers reap the benefits of the food crops that they've planted and nursed during the growing season. This stew comes from a tradition that is hundreds of years old.

INGREDIENTS | SERVES 8–10

5 cups beef, chicken, or vegetable broth

2 medium Yukon gold potatoes, peeled and cut into 1" pieces

3 Roma tomatoes, chopped, reserve the juice

1 cup chopped celery

½ cup chopped green bell pepper

1 small onion, chopped

2 cups shredded cabbage

4 ounces fresh green beans, trimmed and cut in half

1 small zucchini, chopped

8–10 fresh oregano sprigs, tied in a bunch

¼ teaspoon salt

¼ teaspoon freshly ground black pepper

1. In a Dutch oven, add the broth, potatoes, tomatoes and juice, celery, green pepper, and onion. Bring to a boil over medium-high heat.

2. Reduce the heat and simmer uncovered for 15 minutes. Add the remaining ingredients, except the salt and pepper.

3. Simmer uncovered, 15 minutes more, until the vegetables are tender.

4. Remove and discard the oregano sprigs. Season with salt and pepper.

Slow-Cooker Mediterranean Stew

The Mediterranean region is an excellent climate for growing many foods and spices with a high nutrient content. This stew uses slow-cooking methods to extract as many of those nutrients as possible.

INGREDIENTS | SERVES 8

1 medium butternut squash, peeled, seeded, and cubed

2 cups cubed eggplant, with peel

2 cups cubed zucchini

1 (10-ounce) package frozen okra, thawed

8 ounces puréed fresh tomatoes

1 cup chopped onion

1 ripe tomato, chopped

1 carrot, thinly sliced

½ cup vegetable broth

1 clove garlic

½ teaspoon ground cumin

½ teaspoon ground turmeric

¼ teaspoon crushed red pepper

¼ teaspoon ground cinnamon

¼ teaspoon paprika

Combine all ingredients in a 4–6 quart slow cooker and cook on low for 8–10 hours.

Lamb Mediterranean Stew

Start by seasoning 1 pound of cubed lamb with salt and pepper. Heat a sauté pan over medium heat, and add approximately 3 tablespoons of olive oil. When the oil is hot, add the lamb. Sauté until each side is brown, about 1 minute per side, but only long enough to create a light brown crust. Add the lamb to your slow cooker with the other ingredients. Cook until the lamb is fully cooked, about 7–8 hours.

Nikki's Stew

Make your stews spicy to add more heat on cooler days. Add ginger, mint, black pepper, ajwain seeds (available in Indian markets), and cumin to add flavor and aid digestion

INGREDIENTS | SERVES 8

2 medium yellow onions, chopped into bite-size pieces

½ pound red potatoes, chopped into bite-size pieces

½ pound sweet potatoes, chopped into bite-size pieces

4 carrots, chopped into bite-size pieces

3 zucchini, chopped into bite-size pieces

1 yellow squash, chopped into bite-size pieces

Filtered water

Herbes de Provence

¼ teaspoon salt

1. Place the vegetables in a slow cooker with enough water to cover them. Add the herbes de Provence and salt.

2. Cook overnight on low (8–10 hours).

Paleo Version

The Paleo Diet consists of eating fish, chicken, meats, vegetables, some root vegetables, eggs, and nuts. It excludes grains, legumes, potatoes, dairy products, refined sugars, and salts. For a Paleo version of this recipe, replace the red potatoes with butternut squash. Butternut squash has a smooth and sweet taste. For a complete meal, precook some lamb stew meat and add it to the recipe.

Corn Soup

This delicious recipe is courtesy of Chef Priscila Satkoff, Salpicón restaurant, Chicago, Illinois.

INGREDIENTS | SERVES 4

8 cups water, divided

8 medium ears corn, husked and kernels cut off

1 medium white onion

½ teaspoon salt, divided

3 star anises

4 serrano chilies

1. In a stockpot, bring 7 cups of water to a boil. Add the corn kernels, onion, and ¼ teaspoon salt. Reduce heat and let it simmer for about 5 minutes.

2. Remove from heat and let it cool.

3. In a blender, purée the cooked kernels with the onion and remaining water, and strain. Put the soup back into the pot.

4. Boil the star anises with the serranos in a small saucepan over medium heat for 5 minutes. Then add to a blender, and blend the chilies and the star anises. Add ¼ teaspoon salt. Set aside.

5. Bring the corn purée to a boil.

6. Immediately before serving, add a few drops of the serrano and star anise mixture.

CHAPTER 15

Sides

Spiced Sweet Purée
182

Red and Green Gazpacho
183

Summer Chicken Salad
184

Blanched Asparagus or String Beans
.185

Pineapple Slaw
186

Lemon-Basil Green Beans
186

Calabacitas
187

Mixed Vegetables
188

Blanca's Spicy Cauli-Rice
189

Braised Sweet Onions
190

Spicy Okra with Tomatoes
191

Spicy Asian-Inspired Mushrooms
192

Ratatouille
193

Vegetable Curry
194

Spinach with Crispy Shallots
195

Brown Rice with Peas
196

Swiss Chard with Olives
197

Roasted Plum Tomatoes
198

Roasted Carrots
198

Roasted Zucchini
199

Roasted Asparagus
199

Roasted Sweet Potatoes
200

Roasted Pepper Fillets
200

Roasted Corn with Herbs
201

Roasted Peppery Onions
201

Roasted Artichokes and Potatoes
202

Braised Butternut Squash
203

Oven-Baked French Fries
204

Fit Fries
205

Braised Fingerling Potatoes
206

New Potato Salad
207

Baby Red Potatoes with Cilantro
208

Roasted Potatoes with Basil
209

Grated Potato Pancakes
210

Green Brown Rice
211

Baked Brown Rice
212

Brown Rice Polenta
213

Herbed Rice Pilaf
214

Another Herbed Rice
215

Five-Spice Rice
216

Spiced Sweet Purée

This recipe is a healthful way to balance your sweet cravings, and a great Thanksgiving side dish as well.

INGREDIENTS | SERVES 4

5 medium sweet potatoes, peeled and cut into cubes

2 tablespoons olive oil

2 tablespoons ground cinnamon, divided

1 teaspoon ground allspice

½ teaspoon freshly grated nutmeg, divided

4 tablespoons virgin coconut oil

1 teaspoon vanilla extract

1. Preheat the oven to 345°F.

2. Put the peeled and cubed sweet potatoes into a glass 9" × 9" baking pan, drizzle with olive oil and mix, making sure every piece is coated in the olive oil.

3. Sprinkle with 1 tablespoon cinnamon, the allspice, and ¼ teaspoon nutmeg. Mix well to make sure every piece is coated with the spices.

4. Bake for 45 minutes.

5. Mash the sweet potatoes. Add the coconut oil, vanilla, remaining cinnamon, and remaining nutmeg. Mix and serve.

Red and Green Gazpacho

This colorful version of gazpacho makes an excellent appetizer. Use the coolness of this soup to counteract the fiery spices in a meal, or to cool off from the summer heat.

INGREDIENTS | SERVES 8

1 clove garlic, minced

¼ cup chopped green onions

½ cup cucumber, chopped

1 large jalapeño, chopped

4 green tomatoes, chopped

½ cup tomatillo, chopped

2 cups puréed tomatoes

⅛ teaspoon pepper sauce

1 tablespoon tablespoons olive oil

1 tablespoon lime juice

¼ cup cilantro, finely cut

8 ounces medium shrimp, peeled and cooked

1. Add the garlic, onions, cucumbers, jalapeños, green tomatoes, tomatillo, and puréed tomatoes to a large bowl.

2. In a separate bowl, mix pepper sauce, oil, lime juice, and cilantro. Add to the larger bowl with the vegetables, cover, and chill for 1 hour.

3. Chop the cooked shrimp and add to the bowl. Mix and serve.

Tortilla Chip Alternative

Try a plain rice cake. Adding the Gazpacho on top makes a refreshing appetizer during the summer. Try replacing the shrimp with langostino, lobster, or scallops.

Summer Chicken Salad

This summer salad is filled with cool, nutritious flavors that can make any whole foods–based diet a delicious experience. Adding a pinch of cayenne creates a nice mix of coolness and heat.

INGREDIENTS | SERVES 6

1 clove garlic, minced

2 tablespoons extra-virgin olive oil, plus 1½ teaspoons

1½ tablespoons lemon juice, plus 1 teaspoon

1 tablespoon almond oil

¼ teaspoon salt

1 teaspoon dried herbes de Provence

6 cups mixed salad greens

1 ripe mango, peeled, pitted, and diced

2 cups roasted chicken, skinned and chopped

1 avocado, peeled, pitted, diced just before serving

1. In a small bowl or container, combine the garlic, olive oil, lemon juice, almond oil, salt, and herbes de Provence. Shake or stir the dressing well.

2. In a large bowl, toss the salad greens, mango, and chicken. Add the dressing and mix.

3. Garnish with avocados.

Blanched Asparagus or String Beans

Asparagus must be harvested soon after it sprouts, as it can grow up to 10 inches or more in a day. Use fresh asparagus and cook it within a day or two of purchasing or it will harden.

INGREDIENTS | SERVES 6

1 pound asparagus or string beans

1 tablespoon olive oil

1 teaspoon lemon juice

½ teaspoon salt

½ teaspoon freshly ground pepper

1. Blanch the vegetables in a large pot of boiling water for 3–5 minutes, and then chill them in bowl of cold water for 3–5 minutes.

2. Toss with the olive oil and lemon juice. Season with salt and freshly ground pepper.

Excellent Holiday Side Dish

This simple recipe makes a delicious side dish during the holidays. After week 9, add some sliced almonds for a little more texture. You may also add some Bragg Liquid Aminos for a different taste.

Pineapple Slaw

Pineapple provides anti-inflammatory enzymes that help with digestion.

INGREDIENTS | SERVES 8

1 cup diced pineapple, drained

3 cups shredded cabbage

1 cup Homemade Mayonnaise (see recipe in Chapter 11)

1. In a medium bowl, combine the pineapple and grated cabbage.

2. Add the Homemade Mayonnaise and mix. Chill, then serve.

Hawaiian Burger

The Hawaiian Burger is a great way to combine protein and sweetness. Serve your favorite hamburger on a bed of mixed greens with a generous amount of pineapple slaw. After week 9, add some raisins to your slaw.

Lemon-Basil Green Beans

This flavorful combo is a popular staple in Asian dishes. Although best known as an ingredient in Italian cuisine, basil is also used in many Vietnamese recipes.

INGREDIENTS | SERVES 4

¼ teaspoon salt

1 pound green beans

1½ teaspoons freshly grated lemon zest

⅛ teaspoon ground pepper

¼ cup fresh basil, thinly sliced

1. Boil a large pot of water over medium-high heat and add the salt. Add the green beans, and cook them for 5–6 minutes. Remove the beans and place them on a plate.

2. Add the lemon zest, and season with salt and pepper. Add basil for garnish.

Calabacitas

This Mexican-inspired recipe makes an excellent side dish, topping, or filling for omelets. Mix in lime juice, tomatoes, or cilantro to taste.

INGREDIENTS | SERVES 4–6

1 tablespoon olive oil

1 small onion, chopped

½ black pepper

1 jalapeño, chopped

2 pounds zucchini, thinly sliced in half rounds

½ cup frozen corn kernels

¾ teaspoon salt

½ teaspoon chili powder

4 tablespoons water

Calabacitas Scramble

To make a delicious egg dish, add ½ cup Calabacitas to a sauté pan, and warm for about 1–2 minutes. Add 3–4 eggs, season with salt and pepper, and scramble until the eggs are fully cooked. Calabacitas are also delicious as a filling for omelets.

1. In a large skillet, heat the olive oil over medium heat, add the onions, and season with pepper. Cook for approximately 2 minutes or until the onions are soft.

2. Add the jalapeño, zucchini, corn, salt, and chili powder. Stir until well combined and cook for approximately 5 minutes, until the zucchini are softened.

3. Add the water, cover, and cook 2 minutes at low heat, until the zucchini are fully cooked and tender.

Mixed Vegetables

Corn has been a staple in many societies for thousands of years. It is a good source of fiber and antioxidants for eye health.

6 small red potatoes, quartered

3 tablespoons olive oil

1 large onion, diced

2 mild green chilies, seeded, ribbed and chopped

1½ cups corn kernels, fresh or frozen (and thawed)

½ teaspoon salt

½ teaspoon pepper

1 tablespoon fresh cilantro for garnish

1. In a large saucepan over medium heat, boil water and add potatoes. Cook the potatoes in water for 15 minutes or until tender. Drain and reserve.

2. Meanwhile, heat the oil in a large skillet. Add the onion and chilies, and sauté over medium heat until tender and fragrant, about 8 minutes.

3. Stir in the corn, salt, and pepper. Stir in the cooked potatoes.

4. Serve garnished with cilantro.

Blanca's Spicy Cauli-Rice

This spicy dish is a great rice substitute, filled with spices that warm and heal the body. It's perfect for a cold winter day.

INGREDIENTS | SERVES 6

1 medium cauliflower head, chopped
⅓ cup virgin coconut oil
1 tablespoon mustard seeds
¼ teaspoon garlic
1 teaspoon ground ginger
1 teaspoon turmeric
1 tablespoon curry powder
1 teaspoon black pepper
4 green chilies, minced

1. Process cauliflower chunks until they are the size of rice grains.

2. Add coconut oil to large skillet. Add mustard seeds to skillet, and heat over medium heat until mustard seeds begin to pop, about 2–3 minutes.

3. Add garlic, ginger, turmeric, curry, black pepper, and 2 tablespoons cinnamon and cook another 2 minutes.

4. Add cauliflower "rice," green chilies, and remaining cinnamon to pan and stir ingredients well. Cover and cook for another 5–10 minutes until cauliflower softens a bit.

Braised Sweet Onions

Many fruits and vegetables have a higher nutritional value in their peels and outer layers. Onions are no different, so don't peel away too many layers. You could be peeling away some of the benefits.

INGREDIENTS | SERVES 4

3 tablespoons olive oil

2 medium sweet onions, peeled and cut into wedges

½ teaspoon coarse salt

⅛ teaspoon freshly ground pepper

1 cup Chicken Stock (see recipe in Chapter 14)

3 sprigs thyme

3 sprigs rosemary

1. Preheat the oven to 350°F.

2. Add the olive oil to a large nonstick pan and heat over medium heat. Add the onion wedges, and season with salt and pepper. Brown the onions, approximately 5 minutes on each side.

3. Transfer the browned onions to a glass 9" × 9" baking dish.

4. Pour the chicken stock over the onions. Add the thyme and rosemary.

5. Bake the onions for approximately 1 hour until they are tender and the stock is reduced, basting them every 10–15 minutes with the cooking juices.

6. Remove from the oven, and serve. They are a nice side for steak or chicken.

Spicy Okra with Tomatoes

Okra is loaded with beneficial fiber and vitamins that make it an excellent addition to a candida diet plan. The fiber helps keep things moving and feed beneficial bacteria, while the vitamins support healthier immune function.

INGREDIENTS | SERVES 8

1 tablespoon extra-virgin olive oil

1 medium onion, diced

1 teaspoon finely chopped garlic

1 teaspoon finely chopped fresh ginger

1 pound okra, sliced into ¼"-thick rounds

4 cups chopped tomatoes

1 teaspoon finely chopped serrano pepper

1. Heat the olive oil in medium sauté pan on low. Add the onions and cook for 3 minutes.

2. Add the garlic and ginger, and cook, stirring, for about 15 seconds, before adding the okra, tomatoes, and peppers.

3. Cook, stirring often, until okra becomes a little gooey, about 20 minutes. Serve hot.

Spicy Asian-Inspired Mushrooms

This is a delicious mushroom recipe that can be served as a side dish for any main protein, especially baked salmon.

INGREDIENTS | SERVES 4

2 tablespoons olive oil

2 pounds sliced white or cremini mushrooms

2 tablespoons freshly grated ginger

½ tablespoon red pepper flakes

2 tablespoons Bragg Liquid Aminos

1 tablespoon sesame seeds

Mushrooms Are Like Sponges

If you wash or soak mushrooms they will absorb water, like a sponge. This will result in a soggy mushroom. To clean them, use a wet paper towel, and just clean the surface.

1. In a large skillet over medium heat, add the olive oil and let it heat for 1 minute.

2. Add the mushrooms and stir with a wooden spoon for 4 minutes until they start to shrink.

3. Add the fresh ginger and pepper flakes, and cook for 2 more minutes, stirring to make sure all the mushrooms are coated.

4. Finally, add the Bragg Liquid Aminos and stir to coat every mushroom.

5. Sprinkle the sesame seeds for garnish.

Ratatouille

Ratatouille is a good example of French home cooking that has captured the taste buds of people worldwide. Prepare the vegetables in advance, except for the eggplant, which can be done right before you start cooking.

INGREDIENTS | SERVES 10

1 tablespoon olive oil

1 medium roasted onion, cut into medium dice

1 small eggplant, peeled (optional) and cut into large dice

1 red bell pepper, cut into large dice

1 yellow bell pepper, cut into large dice

2 medium zucchini, cut into large dice

1 tablespoon chopped fresh garlic

1 tablespoon dried oregano

4 cups chopped tomatoes

½ teaspoon salt

½ teaspoon pepper

1. Lightly coat a large sauté pan with olive oil and set it over medium-low heat. Add the onions and cook about 10 minutes.

2. Add the eggplant and bell peppers and cook, stirring often, until they begin to soften, about 20 minutes.

3. Add the zucchini, garlic, and oregano, and cook, stirring, for 5 minutes.

4. Add the tomatoes and cook, stirring, until thick and aromatic, about 15 minutes.

5. Season with salt and pepper and serve.

Vegetable Curry

Indian herbs are powerful spices, and turmeric leads the way. Together, they are known to block all cancer pathways and reduce inflammation. An Indian dish with curry is always one of your best bets for a healthier life.

INGREDIENTS | SERVES 8

1 tablespoon extra-virgin olive oil

1 teaspoon finely chopped fresh garlic

1 small onion, diced

4 teaspoons curry powder

2 medium baking potatoes, peeled and diced

2½ cups Vegetable Stock (see recipe in Chapter 14)

¼ teaspoon sea salt

4 cups cauliflower florets

6 medium carrots, chopped

1. Add the oil to large sauté pan and heat over low. Add the garlic, onions, and curry, and cook for 1–2 minutes.

2. Add the potatoes, stock, and salt, and simmer until the potatoes are slightly soft. Add the cauliflower and carrots and cook another 5 minutes. Serve.

Purée

Turn this recipe into a delicious purée, use it as a side dish, or turn it into a soup. Add all the cooked curry to a blender and blend to the desire texture. If you are making a soup, add more vegetable stock.

Spinach with Crispy Shallots

Shallots are a favorite among chefs worldwide. Exported to France during the Crusades, shallots' culinary popularity has continued to increase over the centuries. Like onions, shallots release irritants to the eyes when sliced, but they also have a high vitamin A content that benefits eye health.

INGREDIENTS | SERVES 8

2 tablespoons olive oil
4 large shallots, thinly sliced
1 (10-ounce) package fresh spinach
2 tablespoons lemon juice
½ teaspoon salt
½ teaspoon pepper

1. Heat the oil in large skillet over medium-high until hot.

2. Add the shallots and cook until crisp, stirring often, about 8 minutes. Remove them from the pan.

3. Sauté the spinach in skillet until wilted, about 5 minutes.

4. Add the lemon juice and stir. Drain the spinach, and season it with salt and pepper.

5. Serve the spinach topped with the crispy shallots.

Brown Rice with Peas

This is an easy recipe to whip up and stores well in the refrigerator if you want to make larger portions to reheat or even eat cold. Green peas, green beans, and string beans are three legumes that work well on a candida diet plan.

INGREDIENTS | SERVES 8

2 cups brown rice
Water to cover rice, plus 4 cups, divided
¼ teaspoon sea salt
½ teaspoon ground cumin
1 bay leaf
1 cup frozen peas

Tip

If you usually keep homemade chicken or beef stock on hand, adding the stock to this dish makes your rice even more flavorful. Simply replace the water content in this recipe with chicken, beef, or vegetable stock. After week 9, you may use store-bought stock; just make sure it doesn't include sugar.

1. Place the rice in a large bowl. Add water to cover and let sit for 10 minutes. Drain and rinse.

2. In a large saucepan, combine the rice and water. Stir in the salt, cumin, and bay leaf. Bring to a boil, reduce heat to low, cover, and simmer for about 45 minutes.

3. Stir in the peas and cook for 5 more minutes.

4. Remove the bay leaf. Fluff the rice with a fork and serve hot.

Swiss Chard with Olives

Swiss chard is packed with vitamins A, B, C, and K, as well as several minerals and fiber. It can be cooked in many ways, eaten raw, or juiced. Avoid Swiss chard if you are prone to kidney stones.

INGREDIENTS | SERVES 4

1 teaspoon extra-virgin olive oil

1 small yellow onion, thinly sliced

2 garlic cloves

1 jalapeño, finely chopped

2 small bunches Swiss chard, stems separated, and chopped into 1" pieces

⅓ cup pitted and roughly chopped brine-cured olives

½ cup water

1. In a large pan or skillet, heat the olive oil on medium. Add the onion, garlic, and jalapeño. Cook until the onions are soft, approximately 6–7 minutes.

2. Add the Swiss chard stems and olives; they take longer to cook. Add the water, cover, and cook 3 minutes.

3. Add in the Swiss chard leaves and cover. Continue cooking until the stems and leaves are tender, but not soggy, about 4 minutes.

Roasted Plum Tomatoes

Plum tomatoes are more commonly known as Roma or Italian tomatoes because they make better sauces than other varieties. High in vitamins and minerals, plum tomatoes are a good snack.

INGREDIENTS | SERVES 4

3 pounds plum tomatoes, cut in half, seeds and stems removed
1 tablespoon olive oil
1 tablespoon marjoram or thyme

Roasting Vegetables

Roasted tomatoes are great alone or in salads. Roasting draws out natural flavors while preserving nutrients.

1. Preheat the oven to 400°F.

2. Place the tomatoes on a parchment-lined 9" × 13" baking sheet, cut-side up.

3. Drizzle with olive oil and fresh herbs.

4. Roast for 5 minutes, then reduce the heat to 325°F for 1¾ hours.

Roasted Carrots

A delicious companion to chicken or beef, this dish has a sweet, earthy flavor.

INGREDIENTS | SERVES 4–6

2 pounds carrots, peeled
1 tablespoon olive oil
½ teaspoon salt
½ teaspoon pepper

Roasted Carrot Soup

After the carrots are cooked, put them in the blender. Add some fresh ginger and about 1 cup chicken stock. Blend until thick, then add salt and pepper to taste. Try roasting the ginger with the carrots for a stronger ginger taste.

1. Preheat the oven to 400°F.

2. Peel the carrots and toss them in a 13" × 18" baking pan with the olive oil, salt, and pepper.

3. Roast the carrots for about 35 minutes, turning occasionally, until they are tender and turn an amber brown color.

Roasted Zucchini

Make sure that the zucchini isn't overcooked. Buy zucchini that have a firm texture and supple skin.

INGREDIENTS | SERVES 8

2 pounds zucchini, sliced into 1" pieces
1 tablespoon extra-virgin olive oil
½ teaspoon salt
½ teaspoon pepper

Roasted Squash Medley

Give this recipe a colorful twist and more texture by adding yellow squash to the zucchini mix. Cut the yellow squash into 1"-thick rounds, and combine it with the rest of the ingredients.

1. Preheat the oven to 400°F.

2. Place the zucchini in a 13" × 18" baking pan, and toss them with the olive oil, salt, and pepper.

3. Roast for 10–15 minutes, turning occasionally.

Roasted Asparagus

Asparagus is delicious roasted with coarse salt. It is a highly alkalizing food for the urinary tract. If you have kidney and bladder problems, daily consumption will be beneficial.

INGREDIENTS | SERVES 4

1 pound asparagus
1 tablespoon extra-virgin olive oil
½ teaspoon salt
½ teaspoon pepper

1. Preheat the oven to 400°F.

2. Cut the tough ends off the asparagus.

3. Place them in a 9" × 13" baking pan and toss with the olive oil, salt, and pepper.

4. Roast for 20–30 minutes, turning occasionally.

Roasted Sweet Potatoes

These potatoes are delicious in salads or as a traditional side dish to meats.

INGREDIENTS | SERVES 4–6

2 pounds sweet potatoes, cubed
1 tablespoon extra-virgin olive oil
½ teaspoon salt
½ teaspoon pepper
½ tablespoon herbs such as thyme

1. Preheat the oven to 400°F.

2. Place the sweet potatoes on a 9" × 13" baking dish and toss with the olive oil, salt, pepper, and herbs.

3. Roast about 30 minutes, turning occasionally, until slightly tender.

Roasted Pepper Fillets

Try adding some Indian spices to these fillets to give them superb healing properties. Adding ajowan, also known as carom or ajwain, along with mint gives a cool, spicy flavor.

INGREDIENTS | SERVES 8

6 bell peppers (red and/or yellow)
1 teaspoon chopped fresh oregano
  (optional)
⅛ teaspoon sea salt

Multipurpose Ingredients

Roasted bell peppers are always a great ingredient to have on hand. They make a great addition to mayonnaise, as a topping on your favorite salad or burger. Try adding them to scrambled eggs.

1. Preheat the oven broiler on high. On a 13" × 18" baking pan, roast the peppers until skin is charred slightly, about 10 minutes. Turn once after 5 minutes.

2. Remove and cover with foil, letting cool for 30 minutes.

3. Place under cool running water to peel away the skin. Slice the peppers open and remove the seeds. Slice the peppers into strips.

4. Season with oregano (if using) and salt and serve.

Roasted Corn with Herbs

Roasting ears of corn in their husks adds a smoky flavor.

INGREDIENTS | SERVES 6

6 ears corn

⅓ cup equal parts sage and tarragon sprigs

½ teaspoon salt

⅓ cup extra-virgin olive oil

1. Preheat the oven to 425°F. Slit the husks and peel them back to remove the corn silk.

2. Fold the husks back around the corn. Tuck in a few herb sprigs, a sprinkle of salt, and olive oil.

3. Tie with kitchen twine, and roast them in a large baking pan until tender, about 25 minutes.

Roasted Corn Soup

After your corn is cooked, shave the kernels off the cob. Put the kernels in a blender, add chicken or vegetable stock, and blend until creamy (approximately 1–2 minutes). If needed, add salt and pepper to taste. Serve the soup warm or cold depending on your preference.

Roasted Peppery Onions

Onions are very high in vitamin C and are a great source of fiber and other helpful nutrients.

INGREDIENTS | SERVES 6

3 large onions, cut in half

1 tablespoon extra-virgin olive oil

½ tablespoon kosher salt

1 tablespoon freshly ground black pepper

1. Preheat the oven to 375°F. Place the unpeeled onions cut-side up on a large baking pan. Drizzle olive oil and season with salt and pepper. Bake in the oven until soft, about 45–50 minutes.

2. Remove the onions and allow them to cool. Peel and wrap in plastic wrap or place in a glass container. Refrigerate up to 1 week.

Roasted Artichokes and Potatoes

The artichoke is actually a flower, and like many vegetables, it was thought to be an aphrodisiac.

INGREDIENTS | SERVES 12

3 lemons, divided

12 baby artichokes, pared down to pale green hearts, cut in half

3¼ pounds potatoes, scrubbed and halved lengthwise (small new potatoes, fingerlings, or purple potatoes)

2 tablespoons extra-virgin olive oil

4 teaspoons chopped fresh rosemary, plus sprigs for garnish

2 teaspoons salt

½ teaspoon freshly ground pepper

An Ancient Edible

Did you know that ancient Greeks and Romans consumed artichokes? Artichokes are native to the Mediterranean and were introduced to the United States in the nineteenth century to Louisiana by the French and in the twentieth century to California by Spaniards.

1. Preheat the oven to 425°F.

2. Fill a medium bowl with water, squeeze the juice of 2 lemons into the water. Add the squeezed lemon halves. Add the artichoke hearts to the bowl of water and set aside.

3. Place a large saucepan with 3 cups water over high heat. Add the juice of 1 lemon and the squeezed halves, and bring to a boil.

4. Drain the artichokes, add them to the boiling water, and cook for 3 minutes. Drain and set aside.

5. Place the potatoes in a large bowl with oil, rosemary, salt, and pepper; toss to coat. Add the artichokes.

6. Spread onto two 12" × 18" pans. Do not overcrowd the pans or the potatoes will steam instead of roast.

7. Roast in the oven until tender and browned, 45–55 minutes. Rotate the pans once to ensure even cooking.

8. Remove from oven and serve.

Braised Butternut Squash

Butternut squash is loaded with carotenoids for better eye health, as well as other nutrients that help improve cardiovascular health and blood sugar, while reducing hypertension and inflammation.

INGREDIENTS | SERVES 8

1 tablespoon extra-virgin olive oil

4 cloves garlic, minced

1½ pounds butternut squash, peeled, seeded, and diced

¾ cup Vegetable Stock (see recipe in Chapter 14)

3 tablespoons parsley, chopped

½ teaspoon salt

½ teaspoon pepper

1. Combine the oil, garlic, squash, and stock in a sauté pan and cook over medium heat for 20 minutes, until the squash is tender.

2. Sprinkle with parsley, and season with salt and pepper.

Oven-Baked French Fries

French fries are a great snack to have now and again. Try sweet potatoes for a higher nutritional content and a lesser effect on blood sugar levels.

INGREDIENTS | SERVES 6

1 egg white

1 teaspoon chili powder

½ teaspoon salt

¼ teaspoon black pepper

1 pound baking potatoes, scrubbed and cut into thick fries

Homemade Ketchup

Combine a 6-ounce can tomato paste with 2 tablespoons water and 1 teaspoon dried basil. Add ½ teaspoon salt. Combine all the ingredients in a large bowl and use instead of ketchup. Canned tomato paste can be used at any time during the candida diet.

1. Preheat oven to 450°F.

2. In a large bowl, beat the egg whites until foamy, and then mix in the spices.

3. Add the potatoes and coat with the mixture.

4. Place potatoes on a nonstick large baking sheet in single layer.

5. Bake for 25–30 minutes, until the fries are crispy and browned.

Fit Fries

This spicy version of French fries can warm up any main dish while providing spices that help improve overall health.

INGREDIENTS | SERVES 4

1 large sweet potato
1 large baking potato
1 tablespoon olive oil
½ teaspoon chili powder
½ teaspoon sea salt

1. Preheat the oven to 450°F.

2. Peel and slice potatoes into thick pieces.

3. In a large bowl, combine the potatoes, olive oil, and chili powder, and toss well. Arrange the potatoes on a large baking sheet and bake for 30 minutes.

4. Halfway through, turn the fries over and continue baking.

5. Use a paper towel to remove any excess oil once the fries are done. Sprinkle with salt.

Braised Fingerling Potatoes

The purple fingerling potato is a popular variety in Peru. These small delicious potatoes are an excellent side dish with grilled steak or a salmon fillet.

INGREDIENTS | SERVES 4

4 tablespoons extra-virgin olive oil

1 medium onion, peeled and thinly sliced

1½ pounds fingerling potatoes

½ teaspoon salt

½ teaspoon pepper

3 sprigs rosemary, divided

1 cup Chicken Stock (see recipe in Chapter 14)

1 tablespoon chopped rosemary

1. Add the oil to large sauté pan over medium-high heat. Add the onions and cook for 15–20 minutes.

2. Add the potatoes, salt, pepper, and 2 rosemary sprigs, and cook for 20 minutes, or until the potatoes brown.

3. Add the remaining rosemary and the stock. Cover and simmer for 15 minutes, turning the potatoes occasionally.

4. Uncover and cook off the remaining stock, about 5–8 minutes. Sprinkle with the chopped rosemary.

New Potato Salad

New potatoes are potatoes harvested while they are young and their skins are still thin, making them an excellent choice for salads.

INGREDIENTS | SERVES 4

12 new potatoes

¾ cup Homemade Mayonnaise (see recipe in Chapter 11)

½ teaspoon salt

½ teaspoon white pepper

2 teaspoons snipped fresh dill

2 garlic cloves, minced

1. In a large pot, boil water over medium-high and add the potatoes. Boil the potatoes in their skins until tender, about 15 minutes.

2. Drain, cool, and quarter the potatoes.

3. Add mayo, salt, white pepper, dill, and garlic, and mix together.

4. Serve chilled.

Baby Red Potatoes with Cilantro

These potatoes are cooked and served whole, so select those that are similar in size to ensure that they cook evenly.

INGREDIENTS | SERVES 5

¼ pound small red new potatoes

1 teaspoon coarse salt, divided

¼ cup extra-virgin olive oil

½ teaspoon freshly ground pepper

½ cup loosely packed fresh cilantro leaves, washed well

1. Place unpeeled potatoes in a large saucepan, and cover them with cold water.

2. Bring the water to a boil over high heat, and add ½ teaspoon salt.

3. Reduce the heat to a simmer, and cook until the potatoes are tender when pierced with a fork, 15–20 minutes.

4. Transfer to a colander and drain.

5. Place the potatoes in a large serving bowl. Drizzle with the olive oil, and season with the remaining salt and pepper.

6. Toss with the cilantro leaves just before serving.

Roasted Potatoes with Basil

Discard potatoes that have dark or soft spots, sprouts coming out of the eye, or green under the skins. Always choose firm potatoes and look for a skin that peels easily.

INGREDIENTS | SERVES 5

5 Russet potatoes, quartered into long
  wedges
3 tablespoons olive oil
6 large basil leaves
1½ tablespoons thyme
½ teaspoon salt
½ teaspoon pepper

1. Preheat the oven to 450°F.

2. Place the potato wedges into a large saucepan of cold water and heat over medium-high until the water starts to boil.

3. Place the olive oil in a large frying pan and heat over medium heat.

4. Sauté the potatoes for about 10–15 minutes or until they brown. Add the basil, thyme, salt, and pepper.

5. Put the potatoes on a baking dish or roasting pan, and roast in the oven for another 10–15 minutes, until the sides are crisp.

6. Serve immediately.

Grated Potato Pancakes

Potato pancakes are a quick and easy dish to prepare. Try substituting sweet potatoes or yams for variety. Add coriander, cumin, ginger, and turmeric spices for an injection of flavor and health-promoting properties.

INGREDIENTS | SERVES 6

2 pounds Idaho potatoes, peeled

1 tablespoon extra-virgin olive oil, divided

1 teaspoon salt, divided

1 teaspoon pepper, divided

Just Add Eggs

If the pancakes won't maintain their shape, add 1–2 eggs to the mixture. Eggs work as glue to keep the pancake together—plus they add protein.

1. Use the large holes of a box grater, or the grating blade on a food processor, to grate the peeled potatoes.

2. Remove any excess water by placing the potatoes in cheesecloth or a clean towel and pressing until all the water comes out. This step will create a crispier pancake.

3. Heat a cast-iron griddle or skillet over medium-high, add ½ teaspoon oil and the grated potatoes and press with a spatula for a rounded shape. Season with ½ teaspoon salt and ½ teaspoon pepper.

4. Once the pancake is brown on one side (6–7 minutes), flip it over and add the remaining oil to make sure both sides brown evenly.

5. Season again with remaining salt and pepper. Cook until golden brown, about 6–7 minutes. Serve whole or cut into smaller servings.

Green Brown Rice

Brown rice contains high levels of manganese and selenium to help support immune function. Soaking in water overnight helps remove enzyme inhibitors and makes for a fluffier cooked rice.

INGREDIENTS | SERVES 6–8

2 tablespoons olive oil

1 white onion, cut into ¼" dice

1½ cups long-grain brown rice

1½ cups water

½ cup finely chopped cilantro

1 poblano chili, seeded and chopped

½ teaspoon salt

½ teaspoon pepper

1. To a heated saucepan over medium, add the oil and onions, and cook for 10 minutes.

2. Stir in the rice. Add the water and bring to a boil. Turn the heat to low, and simmer, covered, for 30 minutes.

3. Turn off the heat. Let stand, covered for 10 minutes. Stir in the cilantro, poblano, salt, and pepper. Serve hot.

Arroz con Pollo (Rice with Chicken)

Serve this rice dish with baked chicken. Simply bake a whole chicken and serve a portion on a bed of the Green Brown Rice. Arroz con pollo is popular in Latin America, especially in Peru. Traditionally, the chicken is also cooked in a cilantro sauce.

Baked Brown Rice

Eating a serving of brown rice each day can help lower your risk of diabetes, cancer, gallstones, heart disease, and high cholesterol. Saffron is the most expensive spice in the world; it also provides a long list of health benefits that includes being an effective antidepressant.

INGREDIENTS | SERVES 6

1½ cups long-grain brown rice

1 small onion, chopped

8 ounces ground beef, browned

2 tablespoons extra-virgin olive oil

14 ounces Chicken Stock (see recipe in Chapter 14)

1½ cups water

½ teaspoon saffron threads

Holiday Rice

After week 9, give this recipe a fun and flavorful twist by adding ¼ cup dried raisins. Try adding fresh pineapple cubes for a sweet and savory taste. Don't wait for the holidays to make this recipe!

1. Heat the oven to 400°F. In a large casserole dish, combine the rice, onion, beef, and oil, mixing to coat the rice completely.

2. In a large pot, boil the stock, water, and saffron. Pour the mixture into the casserole dish and cover.

3. Bake the rice mixture for 25 minutes, covered. Bake 15–20 minutes longer, uncovered. Remove the rice from the oven and let cool before serving.

Brown Rice Polenta

Rice has many uses. Cover this recipe with a homemade sauce and enjoy!

INGREDIENTS | SERVES 2

1 medium yellow onion, chopped
2 cloves garlic, crushed
2 tablespoons olive oil, divided
2 cups brown rice cereal

1. In a large sauté pan over medium-high heat, sauté onions and garlic in 1 tablespoon olive oil until lightly browned, about 5–7 minutes.

2. Add this mixture to the prepared cereal.

3. Form into medium-size patties and brown them in a skillet over medium-high heat with the remaining olive oil, at least 5 minutes per side.

Herbed Rice Pilaf

With more than 40,000 varieties of rice to choose from, you could spend a lifetime trying rice dishes. This herbed version combines the healing properties of cilantro and onions to promote overall health.

INGREDIENTS | SERVES 2

1 cup chicken broth
1 cup water
1 cup brown rice cereal
2 tablespoons olive oil, divided
1 large shallot, minced
1 garlic, minced
3 tablespoons minced fresh cilantro or parsley
½ teaspoon salt
½ teaspoon pepper

1. In a medium saucepan, bring the chicken broth and water to a boil. Add the brown rice cereal, reduce to low heat, and cook for 5–8 minutes until creamy.

2. Add 1 tablespoon oil to medium sauté pan, and sauté the shallots and garlic until lightly browned, about 4 minutes.

3. Add this mixture to the prepared rice cereal. Add cilantro or parsley.

4. Form into medium-size patties, season with salt and pepper, and brown in a medium skillet over medium heat with 1 tablespoon olive oil, at least 5 minutes per side.

Another Herbed Rice

This Indian spice–filled brown rice dish can pack a strong anti-inflammatory, heart-healthy, punch to your life.

INGREDIENTS | SERVES 2

1 teaspoon dried onion flakes

½ tablespoon dried celery flakes

2 tablespoons dried parsley

½ teaspoon dried garlic flakes

½ teaspoon turmeric

½ teaspoon sea salt

1 cup chicken broth

1 cup water

¼ teaspoon ground cloves

1 cup brown rice

1 cup chopped scallions

Combine all the ingredients in a rice cooker ad cook for 40–45 minutes or cook on the stove in a large pot with enough water to cover the rice for 45 minutes.

Five-Spice Rice

This recipe uses a Chinese five-spice powder that is a powerhouse of healing benefits. The spices include star anise, cloves, cinnamon, Sichuan pepper, and fennel seeds. The star anise and Sichuan pepper make it a perfect dish to eat if you have a cold or the flu.

INGREDIENTS | SERVES 3–4

1 tablespoon sesame oil

1 cup brown rice

½ teaspoon sea salt

1 teaspoon five-spice powder

1 tablespoon fresh ginger, minced

½ cup chopped scallion

1 cup frozen peas, defrosted

2 tablespoons Bragg Liquid Aminos

1 cup chicken broth

1 cup water

Mix all the ingredients in a rice cooker and cook for 40 minutes or put in a flameproof, covered casserole and bake for 40 minutes at 350°F or until the liquid is absorbed.

CHAPTER 16

Chicken

Marinated Chicken
218

Lemon and Basil Chicken
219

Roasted Chicken with Oregano
220

Tuscan Chicken
221

Tarragon-Lemon Chicken
222

Chicken, Onions, and Tomatoes over Rice
223

Chicken Pizzaiola
224

Chicken Cacciatore with Porcini Mushrooms
225

Caribbean Chicken with Pineapple Salsa
226

Marinated Chicken

Replacing the curry powder in this recipe with baharat spice powder would give this recipe a Middle Eastern flavor.

INGREDIENTS | SERVES 8

¼ cup Bragg Liquid Aminos
1 tablespoon curry powder
1 teaspoon ground ginger
⅛ teaspoon red cayenne pepper
2 tablespoons olive oil
1 teaspoon cinnamon
1 garlic clove, crushed
2 (4-pound) broiler chickens

Cooking Chicken

Whole chickens must be cooked for 20 minutes per pound. When you split the chicken, it cooks faster. When in doubt, check the temperature with a food thermometer. Chicken should have an internal temperature of 165°F.

1. Mix all ingredients together in a bowl, except the chickens.

2. Clean the chicken, remove as much skin as possible, and split the chicken open to lie flat on a roasting pan.

3. Spread the marinade on both sides of the chicken, cover, and refrigerate for 2 hours and up to 1 day.

4. Preheat the oven to 375°F.

5. Bake the chicken for 1 hour and 30 minutes.

Lemon and Basil Chicken

When available, purchase organic, pastured chickens from a local farmers' market. If that's not possible, buy organic, free-range chickens, and then organic-labeled chickens. These varieties come without the antibiotics found in chickens raised in a conventional manner.

INGREDIENTS | SERVES 6

½ cup chopped spring onions

½ cup chopped fresh basil leaves, plus 1 tablespoon for garnish

1 lemon juiced, plus slices for garnish

½ teaspoon coarse salt

½ teaspoon black pepper

6 chicken pieces (can be a combination of legs, thighs, and breasts for approximately 4 pounds of chicken with bones, or 2½ pounds boneless)

3 tablespoons olive oil

Sage: Chicken's Best Friend

Sage and chicken go hand-in-hand. Try adding dried sage powder or fresh sage to your chicken recipes. Sage has been used by many cultures for many centuries for its healing properties.

1. Preheat oven to 350°F.

2. In a large bowl, mix the onions and basil. Add the lemon juice, salt, and pepper, and mix thoroughly.

3. Rub the marinade onto the chicken pieces and place in a well-oiled 9" × 13" baking pan. Drizzle with a little olive oil.

4. Roast, uncovered, for about 30 minutes, depending on the size of the chicken.

5. Garnish with more basil leaves and lemon slices.

Roasted Chicken with Oregano

Pastured and free-range chickens have higher levels of beneficial fatty acids, vitamins, and antioxidants, and have a better flavor and texture. Adding oregano makes this chicken an excellent dish for the candida diet.

INGREDIENTS | SERVES 4–6

1 whole chicken (about 3½ pounds), cut into 10 serving sizes

4 medium Yukon gold potatoes, cut into medium chunks

4 plum tomatoes, cut into medium chunks

4 medium zucchini, cut into medium chunks

1 large onion, cut into medium chunks

¼ cup extra-virgin olive oil

¼ cup fresh oregano leaves, coarsely chopped

½ teaspoon coarse salt

¼ teaspoon freshly ground pepper

1. Preheat the oven to 450°F; place the rack in the upper third of the oven.

2. Combine the chicken and vegetables in a large roasting pan.

3. Add oil, oregano, salt, and pepper, and toss. Arrange the chicken, skin-side up, over vegetables.

4. Roast until the thickest part of the thigh registers 170°F, about 45 minutes. Remove from the oven and serve.

Tuscan Chicken

Rosemary is an excellent herb to include as an antioxidant when cooking meats. Rosemary is also an excellent source of nutrients that help combat candida, cancer, ulcers, arthritis, skin rashes, and memory loss. Serve this chicken with your vegetable of choice.

INGREDIENTS | SERVES 4

¼ cup olive oil

1 pound boneless skinless chicken breasts, cut into ¼" cubes

8 ounces cherry or grape tomatoes

8 ounces mushrooms, sliced

1 cup chicken broth

¼ teaspoon dried rosemary, crushed

¼ teaspoon freshly ground pepper

1. In a large skillet, heat the olive oil over medium.

2. Add the chicken and cook, stirring, for 3 minutes. Add the tomatoes and mushrooms. Cook and stir for 3 minutes.

3. Add the broth and rosemary. Season with pepper. Bring to a boil and reduce heat to low. Simmer, uncovered, until the liquid is reduced and the chicken is tender. Serve.

Tarragon-Lemon Chicken

The tarragon and black pepper in this recipe can aid digestion and may even bring you back for seconds by stimulating digestive juices. Tarragon is known as the King of Herbs and black pepper as the King of Spices, making this a royal feast.

INGREDIENTS | SERVES 4

⅓ cup olive oil

2 tablespoons finely chopped chives

1 tablespoon finely chopped fresh cilantro

1 tablespoon lemon juice

1½ teaspoons dried tarragon, crushed

¼ teaspoon paprika

1 pound boneless skinless chicken thighs

¼ teaspoon freshly ground pepper

1. Place the olive oil in a small saucepan over low heat. Add the chives, cilantro, lemon juice, tarragon, and paprika.

2. Season the chicken with pepper, and grill it on an uncovered grill at medium-high heat (375°F–400°F) until tender (approximately 10 minutes), brushing it often with the olive oil mixture. Or cook it on the stove over medium heat in the olive oil marinade until the chicken is tender and no longer pink in the center, approximately 12–15 minutes. Serve hot or cold.

Chicken, Onions, and Tomatoes over Rice

Demonstrate your creative flair by adding herbs and spices. As it is, this dish contains powerful nutrients and antioxidants, as well as a rich, full flavor.

INGREDIENTS | SERVES 4

1½ teaspoons coarsely ground pepper, divided

¾ teaspoon salt, divided

1 clove garlic, minced

2 tablespoons olive oil

4 medium skinless boneless chicken breasts

2 large onions, sliced

3 medium tomatoes, chopped

2 teaspoons minced fresh ginger

¼ cup fresh or store-bought pesto (basil and olive oil, no cheese or pine nuts)

4 cups brown rice

1. Combine 1 teaspoon pepper, ½ teaspoon salt, and the garlic, and rub the mixture over the chicken.

2. In a 12" skillet, heat the oil over medium. Cook the chicken and onions in the oil for 15 minutes, or until the onions are tender and the chicken is no longer pink. Turn the chicken once and stir the onions occasionally.

3. Remove the chicken and slice it cross-wise into strips. Return the chicken to the skillet with the tomatoes, ginger, remaining pepper, and remaining salt. Heat through.

4. Stir in the pesto, and serve the chicken and sauce on top of the brown rice.

Chicken Pizzaiola

Pizzaiola, a traditional Neapolitan dish, is translated as "Pizza Style." Traditionally, this dish is made with beef and is called Carne Pizzaiola. You can serve it on top of brown rice or spaghetti squash.

INGREDIENTS | SERVES 4

2 tablespoons olive oil, divided

1 large onion, finely chopped

2 cloves garlic, chopped

2 cups freshly chopped tomatoes, reserve the liquid

½ cup chopped basil

1 teaspoon dried oregano, crushed

1 pound boneless skinless chicken breasts

Chicken Fact

Gainesville, Georgia, is the Chicken Capital of the World. In 1961, the city passed an ordinance that made eating chicken with anything other than your hands illegal.

1. In a medium saucepan, heat 1 tablespoon olive oil over medium-high. Sauté the onion and garlic in the oil until tender, about 3 minutes. Add the tomatoes, basil, and oregano. Bring to a boil. Reduce the heat and simmer, uncovered, for 5 minutes or until thickened, stirring frequently.

2. Rinse the chicken and pat it dry with paper towels. Lightly brush it with the remaining olive oil.

3. Gently cook in a large frying pan on medium heat for 3 minutes, and then turn and cook for 3 minutes or until the chicken is tender and no longer pink.

4. Place the chicken on a serving platter and top with the tomato mixture to serve.

Chicken Cacciatore with Porcini Mushrooms

Cacciatore is an Italian word for "hunter." With the antifungal herbs in this dish, candida quickly becomes the prey. Don't be afraid to ask for seconds!

INGREDIENTS | SERVES 4

1 tablespoon extra-virgin olive oil

1 (4-pound) chicken, cut into 12 pieces

½ teaspoon coarse salt

½ teaspoon black pepper

3 garlic cloves, crushed

12 ounces porcini mushrooms, halved

1 medium onion, chopped into small pieces

3 fresh oregano sprigs

3 fresh thyme sprigs

3 medium tomatoes, chopped into small pieces

1 cup Chicken Stock (see recipe in Chapter 14)

1. Warm the extra-virgin olive oil in a large sauté pan on low.

2. Season the chicken pieces with salt and pepper. Brown the chicken in the pan, about 10 minutes, and transfer to a plate.

3. Add the remaining ingredients to the pan and cook for 5 minutes over medium heat. Add the chicken and bring to a boil.

4. Reduce heat to low, cover, and continue to simmer for about 45 minutes or until chicken is thoroughly cooked.

Caribbean Chicken with Pineapple Salsa

Some of the most popular dishes in the Caribbean are served with rice and beans. You can serve this dish with black beans and brown rice starting on week 9. Wait until week 11 to start using white rice.

INGREDIENTS | SERVES 2

CHICKEN

2 cloves garlic, chopped

½ jalapeño, chopped

1 large shallot, chopped

½ cup fresh cilantro

3 tablespoons olive oil

1 teaspoon kosher salt

Juice of 1 lime

2 large boneless chicken breasts

SALSA

1½ cups diced fresh pineapple

3 tablespoons red onion, finely chopped

¼ jalapeño, minced

2 tablespoons cilantro leaves, chopped

1. Purée all the ingredients for the marinade and put it into a zippered plastic bag with the chicken for 30 minutes.

2. Grill the chicken over medium-high heat for 10–12 minutes and serve warm or at room temperature.

3. Combine the salsa ingredients (except the cilantro) and refrigerate up to one day.

4. Add the cilantro to the salsa before serving it with the chicken.

CHAPTER 17

Fish

Marinated Fish
228

Mahi-Mahi with Creole Sauce
229

Scallops á la Adam
230

Baked Tilapia
230

Salmon with Fresh Ginger Sauce
and Rice
231

Barbecued Teriyaki Salmon
232

Grilled Mahi-Mahi
233

Mexican Fish
234

Chesapeake Stew
235

Salsa Tuna
236

Grilled Fish with Salsa Fresca
237

Fish Ceviche
238

Grilled Tiger Shrimp with Two
Sauces
239

Seafood Soup
240

Marinated Fish

Try chopping up the fish, mixing it with a variety of spices, and forming fish cakes that you can cook and eat on top of a rice cake. Substitute 4 tablespoons orange juice concentrate for citrus juice after adding it back to diet in week 9.

INGREDIENTS | SERVES 4

2 pounds snapper, trout, or flounder fillets

1 medium onion, thinly sliced

¼ cup olive oil

1 teaspoon sea salt

¼ teaspoon pepper

4 tablespoons citrus juice (lemon, lime, grapefruit, or any combination)

2 tablespoons Bragg Liquid Aminos

1. Preheat the oven to 350°F.

2. Place the fish on a 9" × 13" greased baking pan.

3. Slash the fish in several places and insert the onion slices.

4. In a small bowl, mix the remaining ingredients. Spread over the fish and baste during cooking.

5. Bake for 20 minutes, or until the fish flakes easily with a fork.

Mahi-Mahi with Creole Sauce

The moist, flaky texture makes mahi-mahi an excellent fish for stews, soups, and main dishes. The seasonings in this dish give it a mild Creole flavor.

INGREDIENTS | SERVES 4

1 tablespoon fresh lemon juice

4 (6-ounce) mahi-mahi fillets

½ teaspoon salt

½ teaspoon black pepper

3 tablespoons olive oil

½ small onion, thinly sliced

½ small red bell pepper, thinly sliced

½ small green bell pepper, thinly sliced

1 medium tomato, chopped into small pieces

1 tablespoon chopped fresh cilantro

1 tablespoon paprika

1 tablespoon extra-virgin olive oil

1. Squeeze the lemon juice over fish. Season with salt and pepper and set aside.

2. Warm the olive oil in large sauté pan over medium, and add the onions and peppers, cooking until slightly tender, about 3–5 minutes.

3. Add the tomatoes and simmer for 8–10 minutes, stirring in the cilantro and paprika.

4. Add the extra-virgin olive oil to a medium skillet, and briefly cook the fish on high, 2–3 minutes on each side.

5. Transfer to a plate and add the sauce.

Scallops á la Adam

This is a simple scallop recipe for those who enjoy their foods without a lot of flair or spices. You can turn this dish into a wonderful healing experience as well by adding ginger, coriander, turmeric, mustard seed, and chili powder!

INGREDIENTS | SERVES 2

Juice of 1 lime
1 garlic clove, crushed
1 pound bay scallops
¼ cup olive oil

Heart Healthy

Scallops are an excellent source of omega-3 fatty acids that have been shown to improve heart health and decrease the effects of stress on the body. Enjoy them weekly and chase your blues away!

1. Mix the lime juice and crushed garlic in a zippered plastic bag. Marinate the scallops in the mixture for 2–3 hours.

2. Add the oil to a medium sauté pan and sauté the scallops over medium heat for 2–3 minutes, or until they are just white.

Baked Tilapia

Tilapia is a good fish for baking because of its sweet flavor and firm, tender textures. Tilapia is a favored fish in many cultures due to its easy availability.

INGREDIENTS | SERVES 2–3

2 pounds tilapia (or any firm whitefish)
2 tablespoons olive oil
¼ teaspoon garlic powder
1 cup chopped cherry or grape tomatoes
3 medium green onions, chopped

1. Preheat the oven to 375°F.

2. Wash the fish and pat dry. Brush with olive oil. Place fish in baking pan. Sprinkle with garlic powder. Place the tomatoes and onions over the fish.

3. Bake 10–12 minutes, or until the oil bubbles. Serve.

Salmon with Fresh Ginger Sauce and Rice

Who says cooking has to be complicated? This simple recipe can be whipped up by even novice cooks.

INGREDIENTS | SERVES 6

Juice of 1 lime

6 (4-ounce) salmon steaks or fillets

⅛ teaspoon salt

⅛ teaspoon black pepper

2 cups Ginger Sauce (see recipe in Chapter 11)

3 cups cooked brown rice

1. Pour the lime juice over the salmon. Season with salt and pepper.

2. Grill salmon on medium-high heat for 4–5 minutes, or wrap salmon in foil and place on a 13" × 18" baking sheet, baking in the oven at 400°F for 20–25 minutes.

3. Serve with Ginger Sauce and brown rice.

Brain Food

Salmon is known for its high content of the omega-3 fatty acid DHA, which has ben shown to be essential for normal brain function and improves mental clarity and brain cell communication. Play around with spices such as chili, saffron, rosemary, sage, and sesame seeds for some additional beneficial brain effects.

Barbecued Teriyaki Salmon

Teriyaki sauce is a great addition to many meat dishes. This basic recipe can be spiced up with chili powder, cardamom, cinnamon, and allspice.

INGREDIENTS | SERVES 6

1¾ cups Bragg Liquid Aminos

⅓ cup grated ginger pulp

1 teaspoon lemon juice

6 (4-ounce) salmon steaks or fillets

6 pineapple slices (freshly cut)

1. Start a charcoal fire 1 hour ahead of cooking time. If using a gas grill, set the temperature at medium-high heat (approximately 325°F).

2. Prepare the teriyaki by mixing the Bragg Liquid Aminos, ginger, and lemon juice in a zippered bag or large bowl. Marinate the salmon in teriyaki marinade for 30 minutes. Discard the marinade.

3. Grill pineapple slices for 1 minute on each side and set aside.

4. Cook the salmon on the grill for 3–5 minutes. Carefully remove from the grill. Serve with the grilled pineapple slices.

Grilled Mahi-Mahi

Along with tilapia and salmon, mahi-mahi is a sustainable seafood choice in most areas of the world. Avoid mahi-mahi from waters around Costa Rica, Peru, and Guatemala, where they are endangered by overfishing practices.

INGREDIENTS | SERVES 6–8

3 tablespoons extra-virgin olive oil

3 tablespoons lime juice

3 garlic cloves, smashed

¼ teaspoon black pepper

3 sprigs thyme

1½ pounds mahi-mahi fillets

1. In a small bowl, combine the olive oil, lime juice, garlic, pepper, and herbs. Add the ingredients to a large plastic bag with the fish. Seal and shake to coat the fish.

2. Refrigerate for 1–2 hours.

3. Remove the fish from the bag and grill or cook in a grill pan over high heat until lightly browned on both sides and cooked throughout, about 2–3 minutes per side. Serve and enjoy.

Mexican Fish

Choose from mahi-mahi, tilapia, halibut, or cod. You can add Salsa Fresca, Salsa Verde, or Pico de Gallo (see the recipes in Chapter 11), or reduce the ingredients to just olive oil, salt, and pepper for more of the natural fish flavors.

INGREDIENTS | SERVES 4

1 cup diced peeled cucumber

1 cup diced red bell pepper

1½ cups diced tomato

½ cup cilantro diced

1 tablespoon extra-virgin olive oil

4 (6-ounce) pieces firm whitefish

½ cup water

1. In a medium nonstick pan, sauté the vegetables on medium in olive oil until they are tender-crisp, about 6–8 minutes. Remove the vegetables.

2. In the same pan, sauté the fish in water on medium until cooked through, about 4–5 minutes for each side.

3. Serve the fish with the vegetables.

Try New Flavors

Experiment with seasonings. Try a little chili powder or lime juice (just a touch) to wake up the flavor in this dish.

Chesapeake Stew

Choose fish that will hold their shape and texture in the broth (red snapper, scrod, halibut), or try adding shrimp, bay scallops, or mussels.

INGREDIENTS | SERVES 8–10

5 cloves garlic, sautéed

2 large green peppers, chopped

1 cup onions

8 cups freshly chopped tomatoes

½ package frozen okra, or 8 fresh okra

1 pound green beans

2 pounds zucchini

8 fresh ears corn, kernels scraped off

12 medium carrots

12 stalks celery

4 cups Vegetable Stock (see recipe in Chapter 14)

1 teaspoon oregano

1 bay leaf

½ teaspoon coarse salt

½ teaspoon black pepper

2 pounds fish (sea bass, flounder, halibut, or other whitefish)

1. In a large pot, combine the vegetables with the stock, herbs, and spices, and cook over medium heat until tender, about 20 minutes.

2. Add the fish and let cook for 5 minutes until the fish is completely cooked and still tender.

3. Remove the bay leaf. Serve in soup bowls.

Salsa Tuna

Prepare the sauce early or the night before to shorten the preparation time.

INGREDIENTS | SERVES 4

¼ cup olive oil

1½ cups diced onions

1 teaspoon red pepper flakes

2 cups diced fresh tomatoes

3 tablespoons puréed garlic

1 tablespoon dry basil

1½ cups diced zucchini

1½ cups diced red bell peppers

¼ cup Salsa Verde (see recipe in Chapter 11)

4 pieces tuna steak, grilled

Tuna Dish Varieties

You can change the color and the taste of this dish by using either the Salsa Fresca or Pineapple Salsa recipes in Chapter 11. For more spice and sweetness, try the pineapple salsa with a tablespoon of chili powder added in.

1. Heat the olive oil in a heavy frying pan and sauté the onions on medium until transparent, about 5 minutes. Add the pepper flakes and tomatoes, and continue cooking until the tomatoes are soft, about 2–3 minutes.

2. Stir in the garlic and basil. Add the zucchini and peppers and continue cooking until they are hot, about 3–4 minutes.

3. Serve ¼ cup salsa on top of each grilled tuna steak.

Grilled Fish with Salsa Fresca

Recipe courtesy of Chef Priscila Satkoff, Salpicón restaurant, Chicago, Illinois.

INGREDIENTS | SERVES 4

2 cups diced plum tomatoes

1 cup finely chopped onion

¼ cup finely chopped cilantro

1 tablespoon finely chopped serrano chilies

2 tablespoons olive oil

2 tablespoons fresh-squeezed lime juice

1 tablespoon extra-virgin olive oil

4 (6-ounce) fish fillets (tilapia, mahi-mahi, red snapper, grouper)

½ teaspoon salt

½ teaspoon freshly ground black peppercorn

1 medium avocado, sliced

Cilantro sprigs for garnish

1. For the sauce, mix the tomato, onion, cilantro, chilies, olive oil, and lime juice in a large bowl. Cover and refrigerate for approximately 1 hour to allow the flavors to marry. Let it warm at room temperature.

2. Rub the extra-virgin olive oil on the fish, and season with salt and black pepper.

3. Cook the fish fillets on a grill over medium heat or in a broiler until they are tender, about 4–5 minutes for the grill and 5–7 minutes for the broiler. Be careful not to overcook.

4. Place the fish on a dinner plate and scoop the tomato mixture on top of the fish.

5. Garnish with slices of avocado and sprigs of cilantro.

Fish Ceviche

Recipe courtesy of Chef Priscila Satkoff, from Salpicón restaurant, Chicago, Illinois.

INGREDIENTS | SERVES 4

½-pound marlin fillets or any comparable firm-textured fish, cut into ½" pieces

5 ounces fresh-squeezed lime juice

1 cup diced plum tomatoes

½ cup finely chopped onion

½ cup finely chopped cilantro

3 serrano chilies or 1 jalapeño, finely chopped

1 tablespoon extra-virgin olive oil

½ teaspoon salt

1 medium avocado, sliced

Cilantro sprigs for garnish

1. Place the fish in a large glass or plastic bowl and pour the lime juice over it (making sure the fish is submerged). Cover and refrigerate for about 4 hours or until the fish has been cooked in the lime juice. Check by cutting a piece of fish; when it shows an even color in the center, it is fully cooked. Strain the pieces of fish.

2. In another large bowl, mix the tomatoes, onions, cilantro, and peppers.

3. Add the cooked fish, olive oil, and salt, and mix.

4. Cover and refrigerate for approximately 1 hour or until it is ready to be served.

5. Scoop the fish into glass bowls or small cups. Garnish with slices of avocado and sprigs of cilantro.

Grilled Tiger Shrimp with Two Sauces

*This is another delicious recipe courtesy of Chef Priscila Satkoff,
Salpicón restaurant, Chicago, Illinois.*

INGREDIENTS | SERVES 4

2 medium avocados, peeled and pitted

2 medium tomatillos (husks removed)

½ cup cilantro

2 cups cold water, divided

¾ teaspoon salt, divided

3 medium plum tomatoes, roasted, peeled and seeded

7 chipotle chilies (seeds removed), soaked in water

1 pound tiger shrimp (16–20 count), peeled and deveined

1 medium fresh mango, peeled and cut into thin wedges

Cooking Shrimp

A handy guideline for cooking shrimp is the shape they achieve from cooking. When the shrimp achieve a "C" shape while cooking, they are considered to be cooked enough. If they are overcooked, they will form into an "O" shape. This tip can help prevent having to eat shrimp toughened from overcooking.

1. In a blender or food processor, blend the avocados, tomatillos, cilantro, 1 cup water, and ½ teaspoon salt to a smooth purée. Set aside.

2. In a blender or food processor, add the tomatoes, chilies, and remaining water. Blend until puréed.

3. Season the shrimp with the remaining salt. Cook on a grill over medium-high heat for 2 minutes each side or in broiler for 2–3 minutes each side.

4. On a medium-size plate, place the avocado sauce on half of the plate, and on the other half, the tomato-chipotle sauce.

5. Garnish the plate with the mango slices and set the grilled shrimp between the two salsas.

Seafood Soup

This seafood lover's dream soup comes to us via award-winning chef Priscila Satkoff, of the Salpicón Restaurant in Chicago, Illinois.

INGREDIENTS | SERVES 4

3 pounds whitefish bones (rinsed under running water until the water is very clear)

1 pound carrots, peeled and cut into pieces

11 garlic cloves

1 stalk celery

2 medium yellow onions

1 tablespoon salt, plus extra to taste

15 guajillo chilies, seeds and veins removed

20 Manila clams

16 New Zealand green-lipped mussels

1 pound monkfish, cut into small pieces

12 ounces fresh calarnari, cleaned and sliced

8 medium-size dry-pack sea scallops

8 medium-size tiger shrimp (13–15 count), peeled and deveined

1 medium onion, finely chopped

10 sprigs cilantro, finely chopped

Juice of 2 fresh squeezed limes

1. Place the fish bones in a large stockpot and cover them with water.

2. Add the carrots, 7 garlic cloves, celery, 1 onion, and salt. Bring to a boil and cook at medium heat for about 45 minutes.

3. Strain and remove the fish bones and leftover vegetables.

4. Put the strained broth back into the stockpot and bring to a boil.

5. Put the chilies in a bowl and cover them with boiling water, letting them soak for 20 minutes or until soft.

6. In a blender, purée the chilies, onion, and remaining garlic, using some of the fish broth; strain.

7. Add the chili purée to the fish broth.

8. Bring it to a boil and let it simmer for 15 minutes.

9. Add salt to taste.

10. Right before serving, in a medium-size pot, heat some of the guajillo-fish broth and add the clams. When they open, remove them from the broth and set aside.

11. In the same broth, cook the mussels. When they open, remove them and put them with the clams. Add the monkfish and cook until tender; remove and set aside with the cooked seafood. Repeat the process with the calamari, scallops, and shrimp.

12. In a warm soup bowl, place the cooked fish and seafood, and add very hot fish broth. Garnish with the chopped onion, cilantro, and lime juice.

CHAPTER 18

Beef and Lamb

Steak Marinade
244

Marinated Beef Tenderloin
244

Marinated Rib Roast
245

Baked Meatballs
246

Beef and Vegetable Rice
247

Mishmash
247

Mexican-Style Chili
248

Picadillo
249

Spicy Beef Chili Without Beans
250

Bowl of Red (Basic Chili)
251

The Perfect Steak
251

Pepper Steak
252

Steak with Basil and Sage Dry Rub
253

Steak with Rosemary and Tomatoes
254

Hamburger or Ground Turkey Hash
255

Cordero en Chilindron (Lamb in Chilindron Sauce)
256

Mustard-Glazed Lamb
257

Lamb Kebabs
258

Beef (or Chicken) Skewers
259

Beef Tenderloin in Morita Chili and Tomatillo Sauce
260

Mexican Meatloaf
261

Long-Simmered Beef Seasoned with Chile Pasilla
262

Grilled Portobello with Chipotle Sauce
263

Steak Marinade

This is a great basic recipe if you want your steak to be the star of the dish.

INGREDIENTS | SERVES 4

½ cup Bragg Liquid Aminos
1 tablespoon garlic
1 teaspoon ground black pepper
¼ cup olive oil
1 (2") piece ginger, minced
2 teaspoons ground coriander
2 pounds flank steak or boneless sirloin tip

1. Combine all the ingredients in a plastic bag or bowl. Marinate the steak for at least 4 hours up to overnight.

2. Preheat the oven to 375°F–450°F.

3. Pan-sear the steaks in a large skillet over high heat, then cook them in the oven for 12–15 minutes.

Marinated Beef Tenderloin

The beef tenderloin, also known as eye fillet, is a very tender cut of beef that works well in marinades.

INGREDIENTS | SERVES 8

½ cup olive oil
½ cup chopped shallots
2 tablespoons chopped fresh rosemary
8 (6–7-ounce) beef tenderloin steaks, 1" thick

1. In a blender, purée the oil, shallots, and rosemary until almost smooth.

2. Pour into a 13" × 9" × 2" glass baking dish. Add the steaks and turn to coat with the marinade.

3. Cover and refrigerate at least 6 hours or overnight.

4. Grill for 3–4 minutes on each side over medium-high heat for medium-rare.

Marinated Rib Roast

The marinating process usually includes an acidic ingredient such as lemon or vinegar. Some recipes call for pineapple juice. The acid helps break down and tenderize the meat. Always try to find a good balance by using herbs, salt, and oil.

INGREDIENTS | SERVES 6

1 tablespoon chopped fresh rosemary
  leaves
1 teaspoon ground black pepper
2 garlic cloves, minced
1½ teaspoons kosher salt
1 (6-pound) beef rib roast
2 tablespoons olive oil

1. Preheat the oven to 475°F.

2. Combine the rosemary, black pepper, garlic, and salt in a small bowl.

3. Put rib roast, rib-side down, in a roasting pan.

4. Rub the roast with the olive oil, and then rub the seasoning mixture on the top and sides.

5. Roast the beef in the lower third of the oven for 20 minutes.

6. Reduce the heat to 350°F and continue to roast until the thermometer registers 130°F, approximately 2 hours (20 minutes per pound).

Baked Meatballs

Baking meatballs instead of frying them saves time and cleanup, and they can easily be added to homemade tomato sauce.

INGREDIENTS | SERVES 6–8

1½ pounds 85 percent lean ground beef

2 free-range eggs

½ teaspoon oregano

½ teaspoon salt

¼ teaspoon pepper

2 tablespoons extra-virgin olive oil

Candida-Friendly Spaghetti and Meatballs

Make your favorite marinara or tomato sauce in a large saucepan, add the meatballs to the sauce, and let them cook for 5–10 minutes over medium heat. Boil or bake a medium-size spaghetti squash. Once the squash is fully cooked, scrape the meat out, and season it with a little olive oil, salt, and pepper. Serve the spaghetti squash warm with meatballs and tomato sauce on top.

1. Preheat the oven to 350°F.

2. Mix the ground beef, eggs, oregano, salt, and pepper in a bowl with your hands.

3. Form the mixture into golf ball–size meatballs.

4. Grease a jelly pan with olive oil, and arrange the meatballs on a jelly roll pan. Bake for 20–25 minutes until the meatballs are browned and cooked through.

Beef and Vegetable Rice

Cooking a large pot of brown rice in advance can make preparing this dish and others even easier. Add vegetables and spices that work with many of the meals you frequently eat.

INGREDIENTS | SERVES 4

1 pound lean ground beef

3 tablespoons Bragg Liquid Aminos, divided

2 cloves crushed garlic

¼ teaspoon ground ginger

1 medium onion, chopped

1 tablespoon extra-virgin olive oil

1 red bell pepper, chopped

3 cups cooked brown rice

1. Add the ground beef to a sauté pan. Add 2 tablespoons Bragg Liquid Aminos, garlic, ginger, and onion. Cook over medium-high for 8–10 minutes or until brown. Drain the excess oils.

2. Add the olive oil, bell pepper, and rice, and remaining Bragg Liquid Aminos, and continue cooking for 5 minutes. Serve warm.

Mishmash

A mishmash is a collection of unrelated things. Here's your chance to let your creativity shine! Play around with single spices or use spice mixes like Chinese five-spice powder, curry, baharat spice powder, herbes de Provence, or make your own.

INGREDIENTS | SERVES 3–4

1 medium onion

1 pound lean ground beef, or ground turkey

Vegetables of your choosing, blanched, grilled, or steamed

4 cups brown rice

1. In a medium sauté pan, sauté the onions on medium for 5–7 minutes.

2. In a large sauté pan, cook the ground beef for 8–10 minutes or until brown.

3. Add the cooked vegetables. Stir to heat and serve over brown rice.

Mexican-Style Chili

Beginning in week 9, add fresh or canned beans into your chili. Adding fresh or canned corn gives more texture.

INGREDIENTS | SERVES 10

2 tablespoons olive oil

5 pounds boneless beef chuck stew meat

2 teaspoons kosher salt

½ teaspoon freshly ground black pepper

¾ cup chicken broth

2 green chilies, diced

3 tablespoons Mexican-style chili powder

3 celery stalks, chopped

4 garlic cloves, minced

1 medium onion, chopped

2 tomatoes, diced

1. In a large skillet, add the oil and cook the stew beef over medium heat for 8–10 minutes or until brown on the outside. Season with salt and pepper.

2. In a 4–6 quart slow cooker, add broth, chilies, chili powder, celery, garlic, onion, and tomatoes. Cook on high for 4 hours.

Picadillo

Picadillo is a traditional dish in Latin countries. Try adding more variety with jalapeños, olives, capers, cinnamon, cloves, and oregano.

INGREDIENTS | SERVES 4

1 tablespoon extra-virgin olive oil

1 pound lean ground beef

½ cup chopped yellow onion, peeled and diced

½ cup chopped green bell pepper, peeled and diced

1 tablespoon fresh garlic, minced fine

1 teaspoon salt

1 teaspoon ground black pepper

1 teaspoon ground cumin

2 large russet potatoes, peeled and diced

2 large tomatoes, peeled and diced

4 cups brown rice

1. Add the oil to a large skillet and cook the ground beef for 5 minutes on medium.

2. Add the onions, bell pepper, garlic, salt, pepper, and cumin. Continue cooking for 5–8 minutes; then add the diced potatoes. Cover, lower heat, and simmer for 45 minutes.

3. Add the tomatoes and simmer for 5 more minutes.

4. Remove from the heat. Serve over rice.

Spicy Beef Chili Without Beans

This is an excellent choice for those who have difficulty digesting beans and therefore never get to experience the joys of chili!

INGREDIENTS | SERVES 4

1 pound lean ground beef, or chopped buffalo or turkey

2 cups chopped organic tomatoes

1 cup corn kernels, organic frozen or organic canned

½ teaspoon chipotle powder

½ teaspoon coarse salt

½ teaspoon black pepper

2 cups cooked brown rice

1. In a large nonstick skillet, brown the beef on medium until it is no longer pink and it crumbles, about 8–10 minutes. Remove the meat, and pour off the drippings. Return the meat to the pan.

2. Add the tomatoes and corn, and heat through. Season with the chipotle, salt, and pepper.

3. Stir in rice before serving.

Week 9 Variation

Legumes are added starting week 9. If you want chili the traditional way, you may use fresh or canned red beans.

Bowl of Red (Basic Chili)

If time allows, cook this chili a day ahead and refrigerate overnight. The cooling and reheating adds flavor.

INGREDIENTS | SERVES 5–6

1 large onion, chopped
3 pounds lean beef
3–4 garlic cloves, chopped or pressed
4 tablespoons ancho powder
4 tablespoons guajillo powder
2–3 teaspoons cumin
3 cups water
½ teaspoon cayenne (optional)

1. In a large cast-iron pot, sauté the chopped onion over medium heat until clear, about 5–7 minutes.

2. Add the beef and lightly brown, about 6–8 minutes.

3. Add the remaining ingredients and stir to mix.

4. For heat, add cayenne to taste.

5. Simmer for 2–3 hours, stirring occasionally. Serve.

The Perfect Steak

Grilling is an excellent way to enjoy steak, especially a New York strip or a similar cut. Meats cooked medium-rare or less have the most nutritional value.

INGREDIENTS | SERVES 2–4

2 (1-pound) boneless New York strip steaks
2 tablespoons virgin coconut oil
½ teaspoon salt
½ teaspoon black pepper

1. Preheat the oven to 400°F.

2. Cover both sides of the steaks with coconut oil. Season with salt and pepper.

3. Sear the steaks in a skillet on high, and then bake in the preheated oven for 5–15 minutes.

Pepper Steak

Adding a little rosemary to meat is an excellent way to counter toxins that can be produced by cooking.

INGREDIENTS | SERVES 2

2 (6–ounce) New York sirloins
2 cups Bragg Liquid Aminos
4 garlic cloves, chopped
1 small knob ginger, sliced
2 medium-size shallots, diced
10 mini sweet peppers, sliced
2 teaspoons cracked black peppercorns
½ teaspoon coarse salt
2 tablespoons extra-virgin olive oil
2 cups brown rice

Sirloin Steak Fact

The New York loin, which is also known as strip loin and Kansas City strip steak, is taken from the short loin of the cow. The muscle that makes up this steak does very little work and therefore is a tender cut of meat.

1. Slice steaks into thin strips and marinate in the Bragg Liquid Aminos for 20 minutes.

2. In a large sauté pan, cook the garlic, ginger, shallots, pepper, and seasonings in the pan with the extra-virgin olive oil for 5 minutes over medium.

3. Add the steaks to the pan and continue cooking for 2–3 minutes.

4. Flip the steaks and cook on the other side for 2–3 minutes.

5. Remove the steaks from the heat and drain off the excess oils. Place the ingredients over a bed of brown rice.

Steak with Basil and Sage Dry Rub

*Basil and sage have double the heart-healthy effect than either one alone,
making their use with meats just what the doctor ordered!*

INGREDIENTS | SERVES 4

3 tablespoons dried basil

1½ tablespoons sage

1 tablespoon kosher salt

1 teaspoon black pepper

4 T-bone steaks, about 1–1½" thick

1. At least 2½ hours and up to 12 hours before you grill the steaks, prepare the dry rub by combining all the ingredients, except the steaks, in a small bowl.

2. Coat the steaks thoroughly with the rub, wrap them in plastic, and refrigerate them until 30 minutes before grilling.

3. Grill over medium-high heat for 2–3 minutes each side for medium-rare doneness.

Steak with Rosemary and Tomatoes

Pan-sear your steaks on high first to lock in the flavor, and then finish cooking them in an oven.

INGREDIENTS | SERVES 4

6 plum tomatoes, halved

12 garlic cloves, halved

¼ cup olive oil, plus 2 tablespoons, divided

1 tablespoon kosher salt, plus ½ teaspoon, divided

2 tablespoons ground black pepper, divided

4 steaks (1" thick)

¼ cup chopped fresh rosemary

1. Preheat oven to 275°F.

2. Combine the tomatoes, garlic, and ¼ cup olive oil in small, ovenproof casserole dish. Season with 1 tablespoon kosher salt and 1 tablespoon pepper.

3. Bake the mixture, stirring occasionally, for 1½ hours.

4. Rub the steaks with a paste made by combining 2 tablespoons olive oil, rosemary, 1 tablespoon pepper, and ½ teaspoon kosher salt about 10 minutes before cooking.

5. Grill steaks 4–5 minutes on each side over high heat for medium rare, or broil for 6–8 minutes in the oven, about 3"–4" from the flame or heat source and serve with warm tomatoes.

Hamburger or Ground Turkey Hash

Start the day with this delicious hash and keep your blood sugar balanced all day long.

INGREDIENTS | SERVES 4

1 tablespoon olive oil

1 medium onion, chopped

1 pound hamburger or ground turkey

1 pound fresh spinach

½ teaspoon salt

½ teaspoon black pepper

3 eggs

1. Heat the oil in a large skillet over medium, and sauté onion until soft, about 7 minutes. Remove from the pan.

2. Add the meat and cook until it loses its pink color, about 5 minutes over medium-high heat.

3. Add the spinach and stir until it wilts, about 2 minutes. Add the onion, salt, and pepper. Remove from heat.

4. In a separate bowl, whisk the 3 eggs.

5. Pour the eggs into the center of the pan and cook slightly before mixing with the rest of the hash, about 2 minutes.

6. Continue cooking until eggs are done, about 2–3 minutes for firm.

Cordero en Chilindron (Lamb in Chilindron Sauce)

This Spanish stew is an excellent way to warm the body and take advantage of the healing properties of black pepper, garlic, saffron, and onion.

INGREDIENTS | SERVES 8

1½ pounds boneless shoulder or leg of lamb, cut into 1" cubes

1 teaspoon salt

1 teaspoon freshly ground black pepper

6 tablespoons olive oil

3 cloves garlic, whole

1 large onion, chopped

4 large red peppers, cored, seeded, and cut into strips

1 cup skinned and chopped tomatoes

2 teaspoons paprika

1 teaspoon saffron powder

1 chili pepper, seeded and chopped, or dried chilies

8 each of green and black olives

1. Sprinkle the meat with the salt and pepper.

2. Heat the oil in a flameproof casserole or large frying pan with the garlic cloves over medium-high heat.

3. Add the meat and fry until evenly browned, about 3–4 minutes. Remove the meat and set it aside. Discard the garlic, if a milder flavor is preferred.

4. Add the onion and peppers to the pan and sauté until they start to soften, about 7 minutes.

5. Add the tomatoes, paprika, saffron, and chili pepper. Return the meat to the pan, cover, and simmer for about 1 hour or until the meat is tender. Add the olives about 10 minutes before serving.

6. Transfer to a heated serving dish and serve immediately.

Mustard-Glazed Lamb

This is a good way to season lamb and fight off a cold or flu. Allspice, chili powder, black cumin, ginger, and turmeric also go well with mustard.

INGREDIENTS | SERVES 8

1 teaspoon dry mustard

1 tablespoon Bragg Liquid Aminos

1 clove garlic

⅛" slice gingerroot, minced

1 teaspoon crushed dried rosemary, or 2 tablespoons fresh rosemary

¼ cup olive oil

4-pound lamb shoulder, leg of lamb, or lamb chops

1. In a small bowl, combine the mustard, Bragg Liquid Aminos, garlic, ginger, and rosemary.

2. Gradually whisk in the olive oil.

3. With a brush, coat the lamb thickly and evenly, and refrigerate for at least 3 hours or overnight.

4. Preheat the oven to 350°F.

5. Roast the lamb in the oven on a rack for 25–35 minutes.

Lamb Kebabs

You can make a vegetarian version with thick slices of squash, onion, bell peppers, eggplant, and mushrooms instead of the lamb.

INGREDIENTS | SERVES 6

Bamboo skewers
1½ pounds ground lamb
1 teaspoon ground cumin
⅛ teaspoon cayenne red pepper
⅓ cup chopped fresh cilantro
2 cups cooked brown rice
Dill for garnish

History of Kebabs

Kebabs originated in the Middle East. Traditionally, small pieces of meat, chicken, or lamb are marinated and cooked over an open flame. In some cultures, the kebabs are served over rice, accompanied by grilled tomatoes, peppers, and yogurt sauce.

1. Presoak the bamboo skewers in water for 20 minutes.

2. Mix the lamb, cumin, cayenne, and cilantro in a large bowl. Let sit in refrigerator for at least 2 hours.

3. Shape the mixture into an oval.

4. Skewer 2–3 ovals on each bamboo stick and grill over an open flame for 4–5 minutes.

5. Serve with brown rice and fresh dill for garnish.

Beef (or Chicken) Skewers

Skewers and kebabs are fun alternatives to conventional cooking methods. Try cutting chunks of fruit and skewering them as well for a new dessert.

INGREDIENTS | SERVES 4

½ cup Bragg Liquid Aminos
2 tablespoons lemon juice
1 clove garlic
½ teaspoon ground ginger
2 tablespoons olive oil
2 medium green onions, finely chopped
1 pound beef sirloin, thinly sliced, or boneless chicken breasts

1. Combine all the ingredients in a large bowl. Thread the meat onto bamboo skewers that have been soaked in water for 30 minutes.

2. Marinate at least 3–4 hours or overnight.

3. Grill on high heat for 8–10 minutes or broil for 12–16 minutes. Broil or grill until the meat is cooked through.

Hot and Creamy Skewer Dip

A delicious dip makes skewers or kebabs even more enjoyable. Combine 1 jalapeño with 1 cup Homemade Mayonnaise (see the recipe in Chapter 11) in a blender. Blend until creamy, adding salt and pepper if needed.

Beef Tenderloin in Morita Chili and Tomatillo Sauce

Recipe courtesy of Chef Priscila Satkoff, Salpicón restaurant, Chicago, Illinois.

INGREDIENTS | SERVES 6

1 cup water
3–4 morita chilies
¼ cup virgin olive oil
1 pound shiitake mushrooms, sliced
2 pounds roasted tomatillos
1 teaspoon salt, divided
6 (8-ounce) center-cut beef tenderloin
 fillets
½ teaspoon fresh black pepper
Chopped cilantro for garnish

1. In a small saucepan, bring the water to a boil over medium. Add the chilies and let simmer for about 5 minutes. Set aside to cool.

2. Add the oil to a medium sauté pan, and sauté the shiitakes for 2–3 minutes over medium-high heat. Set aside.

3. In a blender or food processor, blend the tomatillo and chilies together using some of the leftover water from the saucepan.

4. In a medium saucepan, bring to a boil the tomatillo purée and season it with ½ teaspoon salt. Add the sautéed mushrooms and let simmer over low heat for about 8 minutes; taste and add ¼ teaspoon salt if necessary.

5. On a very hot grill, place the beef fillets, add ¼ teaspoon salt, and fresh pepper, and grill about 6 minutes per side for medium-rare (depending on thickness).

6. On a dinner plate, set the beef in the center and surround with the shiitake sauce.

7. Drizzle the additional sauce over the fillet. Garnish with the chopped cilantro.

Mexican Meatloaf

Courtesy of Chef Priscila Satkoff, Salpicón restaurant, Chicago, Illinois.

INGREDIENTS | SERVES 4

4 tomatillos

¼ medium yellow onion

3 garlic cloves

1 pound fresh ground meat, a beef-veal combination

1 tablespoon salt, plus ½ teaspoon, divided

2 hard-boiled eggs, peeled and cut into quarters

1 large carrot peeled, cut into quarters, and cooked

½ cup peas, cooked

20 haricot vert, cleaned and blanched

Bouquet garni

4 serrano chilies, roasted

6 plum tomatoes, roasted

1. In a blender, blend the tomatillos, onion, and garlic, using just a little bit of water, to make the salsa.

2. Incorporate the salsa with the meat, mix, and add 1 tablespoon salt.

3. Spread the meat in one layer on a wet 12" × 16" cheesecloth (or white napkin). Distribute the eggs, carrot, peas, and haricot vert over the meat.

4. Carefully roll up the meat using the cheesecloth, tying it with kitchen string every 4".

5. In a large stockpot, bring water to a boil. Add ¼ teaspoon salt, the bouquet garni, and the rolled-up meat and boil for about 30 minutes.

6. Take the meat out of the water, unwrap it, and slice into 1" pieces.

7. In a blender, purée the chilies with a little bit of water. Add the tomatoes and blend a little until you get a coarse sauce. Add ¼ teaspoon salt.

8. Top the sliced meat with the salsa. Serve hot or at room temperature.

Long-Simmered Beef Seasoned with Chile Pasilla

This recipe makes use of a little-known fruit common to Mexico and Central America—the chayote. The chayote is like a cross between a pear and a squash and is packed with vitamin C and protein. Recipe courtesy of Chef Priscila Satkoff, Salpicón restaurant, Chicago, Illinois.

INGREDIENTS | SERVES 4

5 quarts water

2 pounds beef brisket, cleaned and trimmed, cut into 2" × 2" dice

1 medium yellow onion

8 garlic cloves, divided

4 sprigs fresh thyme

1 tablespoon salt, plus ¼ teaspoon, divided

10 pasilla chilies, deveined and seeds removed

2 small chayotes, peeled and cooked

1 pound haricot vert, cleaned and blanched

4 medium carrots, peeled, split lengthwise into quarters, and then cut in half, cooked

1 medium zucchini, split lengthwise into quarters, and then cut in half, cooked

1 medium ear corn, cut into thirds and cooked

Juice of 2 freshly squeezed limes

1. In a large stockpot, bring the water to boil. Add the beef, onion, 4 cloves garlic, thyme, and 1 tablespoon salt. Cook for about 1½–2 hours over low heat or until the meat is tender.

2. Take the meat out of the broth, and remove the onion, garlic, and thyme.

3. Put the meat back into the broth and bring to a boil.

4. In the meantime, quickly roast the pasilla chilies in a very hot skillet. It will take fewer than 20 seconds.

5. In a blender, purée the chilies and 4 cloves garlic, using some of the meat broth.

6. Add the chili purée to the meat and broth. Bring it to a boil and let it simmer for 10 minutes over low heat. Add ¼ teaspoon salt.

7. Place the cooked meat in a soup bowl. Add some of the broth and the cooked vegetables. Add lime juice and serve.

Grilled Portobello with Chipotle Sauce

*With more potassium than a banana and a steak-like flavor and texture,
the portobello mushroom is an excellent showcase for the cooking talents of
Chef Priscila Satkoff, Salpicón restaurant, Chicago, Illinois.*

INGREDIENTS | SERVES 4

3 medium plum tomatoes, roasted

2 chipotle chilies, deveined and soaked in water

1 cup cold water

¼ teaspoon salt

½ medium pineapple, diced into small pieces

1 medium jicama, peeled and julienned

1 bunch cilantro, washed, stemmed and chopped

4 medium portobello mushrooms, cleaned and stems removed

Sprig of cilantro for garnish

1. In a blender or food processor, blend the tomatoes, chipotle chilies, water, and salt, until you get a smooth purée. Strain.

2. In a medium-size bowl, mix the pineapple, jicama, tomato-chipotle sauce, cilantro, and salt to taste.

3. On a hot grill, grill the mushrooms for about 5 minutes, flip them, and cook on the other side for another 3–4 minutes.

4. On a medium-size plate, place the grilled portobello, spoon the pineapple mixture over, and garnish with more salsa and a sprig of cilantro.

CHAPTER 19

Beverages

Anytime Lemon-Basil Water
266

Cinnamon-Infused Coffee
266

Digest Tea
267

Spa Water
268

Long-Life Tea
269

Anytime Lemon-Basil Water

Soaking fruits and vegetables in distilled water will give you a refreshing drink. Experiment with herbs and spices as well to create your signature drink.

INGREDIENTS | SERVES 6–8

3 lemons, sliced
1 lime, sliced
1 cup packed basil leaves
½" knob of ginger, freshly grated
12 cups distilled water

1. Place the lemons, limes, and ginger in a large pitcher.

2. Rub the basil leaves between your hands and add to the pitcher. Add the distilled water and refrigerate for 1 hour. Flavors will release into the water.

Week 9 Variation

Give this recipe a sweet taste by adding some watermelon cubes. Try smashing some of the watermelon cubes to add the juice to the water. You can replace the basil with fresh mint as well.

Cinnamon-Infused Coffee

Cinnamon is a sweet, spicy way to add flavor to coffees and other drinks, and it also helps balance blood sugar.

INGREDIENTS | SERVES 2

1 cup water
1 cinnamon stick
2 cups freshly brewed coffee
1 teaspoon cinnamon powder

1. In a small pot, boil 1 cup water with the cinnamon stick. Let cook for about 10 minutes, until the water is light brown in color, and the water content has reduced almost by half.

2. Combine the brewed coffee and the cinnamon-infused water.

3. Serve in a cup and sprinkle the cinnamon on top.

Cinnamon Tea

Try the same method to make cinnamon tea. Just add more water, maybe 2 cups, and an extra cinnamon stick. After week 15, add some honey for sweetness. You may also use this water to make oatmeal after week 11.

Digest Tea

This tea is infused with the digestive healing and soothing properties of ginger, ajwain (carom seeds), and mint. Drink as a hot or iced drink, or add it to other drinks. Try adding other digestive spices like black pepper, coriander, and cardamom.

INGREDIENTS | MAKES 1 QUART

½ cup ajwain seeds

10 mint leaves

1 (3") piece ginger, peeled and sliced thinly

8 cups purified or distilled water

Lemon slices for garnish

Ajwain Seeds

Ajwain are more commonly found in Indian groceries than anywhere else. The seeds can also be chewed to soothe the stomach or aid in digestion. It's common to experience a little heating sensation from these seeds when chewing them for the first time.

1. In a medium sauté pan, lightly brown ajwain seeds over medium heat for 4–5 minutes and set aside. Be careful not to burn them.

2. Crush the mint leaves with a mortar and pestle.

3. Add the seeds, ginger, mint, and water to a large pot and bring to a boil over medium-high.

4. Turn off the heat, and let steep, covered, for 15–20 minutes.

5. Allow to cool and store in fridge. Serve 1–3 teaspoons per cup of tea or hot water, with a slice of lemon.

Spa Water

This is a favorite water served at spas everywhere, but you don't have to go to a spa to enjoy it. Keep this water in the fridge and enjoy it throughout the week.

INGREDIENTS | MAKES 1 GALLON

1 large lemon, sliced thinly

2 limes, sliced thinly

1 cucumber, sliced thinly

3 sprigs rosemary

20 mint leaves

1 (3") piece ginger, peeled and sliced

Add the ingredients to a gallon-sized glass pitcher to soak overnight in the refrigerator.

Green Sun Tea Variation

Add some additional flavor to this recipe by making some sun tea using green tea. Add the ingredients to the sun tea and store in the fridge. You'll be in antioxidant heaven!

Long-Life Tea

Drink this tea every day to help you live a long, disease-free life. The coconut oil and black pepper increase the effectiveness of the other herbs. Use virgin coconut oil in its solid state in this recipe. If the oil is liquid, cool it in the refrigerator just enough to slightly harden the liquid. Don't spill this tea on your clothes or carpet, as turmeric stains!

INGREDIENTS | SERVES 6

2 tablespoons virgin coconut oil

3 teaspoons turmeric powder

½ teaspoon black pepper

½ teaspoon cinnamon powder

¼ teaspoon cardamom powder

¼ teaspoon allspice

¼ teaspoon ginger powder

Lemon slice (optional)

Mint leaves (optional)

1. Place the ingredients in a cup and mix thoroughly. Add lemon slice or mint leaves.

2. Store in a cool place. Do not store in the refrigerator, as it will harden too much and will need to be thawed. Use 1–2 teaspoons in hot water as a tea.

Tea Variations

Try adding a little chili powder or cayenne to this for some added heat. In week 15, you can use raw honey for added sweetness and health benefits, or use the honey as a base in place of the coconut oil.

APPENDIX A

FAQ about Candida

Will a standard blood test help uncover blood sugar problems that might be associated with candida?

The standard blood test is a very poor indicator of blood sugar regulation. It is an isolated moment in time. This is typically true for all the other blood values in standard tests as well. The gold standard for blood testing is the Oral Glucose Tolerance Test. This test will determine how well your body can regulate sugar in the form of glucose, which is the common form found in the body. After a technician takes a baseline reading of your blood sugar, you are given a solution of glucose to drink, and then retested every thirty to sixty minutes over a three-hour period to see how well your body processes the sugar. Most labs will check every sixty minutes. One criticism of this test is that the blood should be checked every fifteen to thirty minutes for a better assessment of how well your body is handling the sugar load. This is more likely to detect fluctuations that might not appear when checking every sixty minutes. The test is usually done to check for prediabetes, diabetes, or gestational diabetes.

A functional assessment of blood sugar regulation is based on this observation. If you feel weak, moody, irritable, fatigued, crave sugars, or have some other difficulty when going too long without food, you may have reactive hypoglycemia (low blood sugar). If you get tired after eating a meal, you may have insulin resistance (high blood sugar). This assessment tends to be just as accurate, or more accurate than the blood tests, as it is a real-life assessment of how well your body processes foods. If either low or high blood sugar is present, following the Blood Sugar Protocol for four months can help create more healthful blood sugar levels.

What is the Blood Sugar Protocol?

The Blood Sugar Protocol is used for cases of high and low blood sugar to help support normal levels of blood sugar.

How many bowel movements should I have each day?

According to medical physiology textbooks, the average number of bowel movements each day should be three to four. Most people seem to have an average of one bowel movement a day. This can increase the body's toxic load and the levels of inflammation within the intestinal tract and elsewhere.

Increased levels of inflammation can lead to Crohn's disease, inflammatory bowel disease, and cancer.

How can I keep my bowels moving more regularly?

Several common approaches range from commercially available laxatives to herbal laxatives and trace minerals. Commercial laxatives contain a chemical that irritates the intestinal tract, which causes an increase of water into the intestinal tract in an attempt to flush out the irritant. Herbal laxatives work via the same principle, but with an herbal irritant and usually other herbs that may help soothe the intestinal tissues. Concentrated trace mineral formulas, such as Trace Minerals Concentrate, gently pull excess water into the intestinal tract without causing irritation. In cases where chronic inflammation is already present, the trace minerals approach doesn't cause any additional irritation. A bulking agent like psyllium is another option; it can help stimulate intestinal contractions that move waste materials out of the body.

May I continue taking nutritional supplements when following a candida diet?

Many patients take numerous supplements, but they may not be of any particular benefit due to inefficient absorption from an inflamed and imbalanced digestive tract as a result of candida and past antibiotic use. For many people, these expensive supplements are just passing through the digestive system and the nutrients are not being absorbed. While they aren't harmful, they aren't particularly helpful either. If you have felt benefits from taking certain supplements, then you may want to continue doing so. If you're not sure, then you can probably do without the supplements for the time being. As you progress through the plan and restore balance to your digestive tract, you'll be able to absorb more nutrients from your foods, as well as any supplements that you may be taking.

Is it possible to sweat too much?

A good rule to keep is everything in moderation. Work your way up to longer sweating sessions, if you're not used to sitting and sweating in a sauna, hot tub, bath, or steam room. As long as you drink plenty of water and replace any minerals you may have lost during sweating, longer sessions should be fine. Listen to your body's feedback and use common sense. Although a hot bath or a dry sauna is the form of sweating most recommended on the plan, it is much more important to sweat any way you can—sauna, hot bath, steam room, hot tub, Bikram yoga.

Do you recommend exercise as a part of the diet plan?

Exercise is good for body, mind, and spirit. It's best to engage in some form of mild to moderate exercise on a daily basis. Excessive exercise can suppress the body's immune system. Sweating associated with exercise is not the same as sweating in a sauna or hot bath. Many people attempt to substitute exercise for the hot baths or sauna and soon complain of cold and flu symptoms.

People usually become more active when they feel better, and because virtually every health-care professional believes that exercise is part of a healthful lifestyle, almost all customers eventually incorporate some form of exercise into their lives. When you choose an exercise activity, make sure it is something you enjoy. As you probably know, good intentions are not enough to keep you involved in an exercise program that you dislike or that is just too dull to keep you motivated.

I sweat a lot when I exercise. Does this count toward my sweating?

Many people believe that sweating is sweating. Exercise sweating doesn't create enough deep-core heating of the body. Also, during exercise, the muscular contraction causes a back-flushing of toxins, so you don't get an efficient detoxification. The plan states that you should sweat six times per week through a sauna, hot bath, steam room, or hot tub.

Those who have tried to accomplish sweating through exercise wind up with the symptoms that are typical of a die-off reaction, which can generally look like a cold or flu, with symptoms of lung and sinus congestion, sore throat, and fatigue.

Should I take medications while following a candida diet plan?

Do not stop taking any medications on your own, without appropriate advice from your health-care provider. Many patients are able to eliminate certain medications or decrease the dosage after they have completed the plan because various symptoms and health complaints have disappeared. The plan tends to help the body function more efficiently, and so the body absorbs and uses the nutrients from foods more effectively; this also applies to medications. Work with your doctor if you need to adjust your dosages accordingly. In addition, the plan leads to improvement in your body's detoxification processes so patients often report fewer and less severe side effects from medications. Ideally, your primary health-care provider will note that prior health problems are alleviated and, therefore, medications are unnecessary and, eventually, the bottles of prescription medications that have become a part of your life become a thing of the past.

Can vegetarians and vegans do the candida diet plan?

Yes. Many vegans and vegetarians have done the plan very successfully. Eat a well-balanced variety of foods and snacks to nourish your body and to truly benefit from the plan. As an addition to the diet, take a good amino acid supplement to ensure that all protein requirements can be met.

Do I have to eat all the foods on the Yes list?

No, eat only the foods that you know work for your body. There are plenty of healthful wholesome foods to choose from!

Do I need to be concerned about minerals?

In today's world, most foods are deficient in minerals due to current farming practices. Additionally, daily sweating sessions can deplete minerals. If you are susceptible to this, take a supplement with trace minerals.

Does my diet need to be restricted after completing the diet plan?

Your diet needs to be considered in terms of foods that support health and foods that do not. Many commonly eaten foods do nothing to contribute to greater health (at best) or to amplify poor health. Ask yourself if the foods you are eating give you the experience of healthy living that you want. If not, change your approach to how you eat.

Generally, foods that need sauces are of a lower quality and devoid of nutrients. Organic whole foods are the best choice. Eat foods that work best for your body in promoting health.

Why is pork not allowed?

Every pork cell contains a virus called porcine endogenous retrovirus. Pork also produces other unhealthy effects in the body. Ingesting pork while your body is undergoing the cleansing process would undermine the effectiveness of the plan. Remember, all other meats (beef, chicken, turkey, buffalo, ostrich) and fish are allowed.

How much water do I need to drink, and what type?

Remember to drink one quart of water for every fifty pounds that you weigh each day, or as close as you can get. If you're not used to drinking enough water, gradually work your way up to the right amount. Any good filtered water works well with the diet to help flush out toxins. Reputable bottle water companies include Fiji, Volvic, and Arrowhead. The number and quality of purified waters has increased in recent years. Reverse-osmosis water is a good option for home water-filtration systems.

I have high cholesterol. Is this diet okay for me to do?

Yes. In general, people obtain good results in this area.

I have multiple sclerosis and am concerned about sweating. Should I be?

This is a frequent question. Many people with MS have followed the candida diet plan successfully. Like anything new, if you're not used to sweating, then you have to work up to it. The skin is the body's largest detoxification organ. Not using it can slow detoxification of the entire body. If you decide to go ahead with the plan, get used to the sweating beforehand. Start slowly.

I hear a lot about candida these days. What is it?

Candida albicans is a form of yeast that lives in everyone. If there is a healthy balance of "good bacteria" in your body, the candida stays in its normal yeast form. If not, it can mutate into a different pathogenic, problematic fungal form, which is detrimental to your health. Since the introduction of antibiotics in the late 1940s, there have been more than 52,000 research studies done on *Candida albicans* and the many problems, conditions, and diseases that it causes in the body.

What do I do if I feel faint in a hot bath?

Place a cold cloth across the back of your neck. Drink cool water. Don't overdo it. Gradually work your way up to sweating.

I've heard friends talk about other diets and feeling worse before they feel better. Does that happen with a candida diet?

This is sometimes also called "die-off" in reference to any detoxification process that pushes out toxins. If your body is already toxic, the body gets overloaded and you may experience symptoms such as lethargy and headaches. People detoxify at different rates, so symptoms, if any, vary greatly.

Can children do the candida diet plan?

Yes, children ages 4 and older are able to do the diet. The dosage for all the supplements remains the same, except the undecenoic acid should be 250 mg twice a day, instead of three times.

Is the sweating on the plan safe for children?

Yes. The sweating protocol for children age 4 and older is the same as for adults. As for adults, if at any time you feel dizzy, nauseous, or faint, place a cool cloth on the back of your neck or step out of the heat to cool off.

I want to keep feeling this healthy. How soon can I repeat the diet plan?

To maintain optimum health and prevention, you should repeat the plan once a year. You can do the plan more often than that if you find a need for doing so.

Do I have to add foods back in after week 8?

No, many people do so much better on a whole-foods diet that they often choose not to return to old eating habits and all that goes with them.

I'm breastfeeding. Is the diet safe for my baby and me?

Patients who have been breastfeeding have successfully and safely completed the diet plan. The supplements have worked well for pregnant and nursing mothers alike and don't create imbalances within the body.

Is it okay to follow the candida diet during pregnancy?

Most studies have shown that saunas and hot baths are safe in uncomplicated pregnancies. Many studies originate out of Finland where sauna bathing is a centuries-old tradition. With a population of just over 5 million, Finland has over 1.6 million home saunas, almost one for every home. Germany, another good source of studies, has over 1.5 million saunas in homes. Only in America are people phobic about sweating. There was a study that showed that elevated temperatures over a twenty-four-hour period could induce neural tube defects. Neural tube defects take place between the third and fourth weeks of pregnancy. This was most likely due to an infection and a fever in that study ("Maternal Fever and Neural Tube Defects"). Several studies show that sustained fevers over the course of a day or more can be potentially problematic, but even then, defects are rare. Effects from these are more likely due to the infectious agent combined with the fevers. Infections can stimulate a specific type of immune response that the body tries to avoid during pregnancy.

On a candida diet plan, you need to sweat about ten minutes, six days a week. That's a long way from a twenty-four-hour elevation of temperature, even when adding the six days together. Additionally, most women are past their fourth week when they find out that they are pregnant. It's up to the woman to decide.

Is it okay to fast while following the diet?
It's not recommended, as the body requires a lot of energy to run its detoxification pathways.

Shortly after starting the candida diet, my menstrual flow was heavier than normal. Is this okay?
The menstrual cycle may have some changes because the body is flushing out toxins. In some cases, old dead tissue that is bound to the uterine wall is sloughed off. Women may be surprised when this happens, but it is just a natural part of the body's detoxification process.

Is there a best way to reintroduce foods beginning in week 9?
Yes. Eat a small amount of the food on the week you are supposed to add in. Wait for three days to see if you have any reaction. Add one food at a time to determine if it is creating a reaction. A common sign of food allergies will be an increase in your body's production of clear mucus. Chemicals can also create the same type of response.

Remember to listen to your body's feedback. A common result of doing the diet plan is a better feedback system that communicates effectively about what works and what doesn't. Many processed foods contain substances that are problematic for the body. Wheat, corn, soy, nuts, and processed dairy are all common allergens. Many people eliminate lifelong allergies to whole foods as a result of following the diet. Allergic responses to processed, industrialized foods are typically appropriate body-based responses that help us avoid substances that can be counterproductive to a healthier body in the long run.

Will the sweating affect my blood pressure?

Occasionally high blood pressure is lowered to normal ranges when people follow the diet plan. Several studies have been done which support the same conclusion, as well as an overall improvement in cardiovascular health. Some people have reported that when beginning the sweating in a hot bath, they felt as though their blood pressure initially increased a little and then decreased again as they accustomed themselves to sweating in the hot bath. Studies show the same result. A good practice is to make sure that you keep yourself well hydrated and drink water while sweating. Avoid excessive heat and prolonged exposures.

How old can you be and start the diet plan?

The oldest person to do the diet was 95 and the youngest was 3½.

What's the best time of the year to do the diet?

There's never a good time to do the diet plan for one reason or another: holidays, birthdays, anniversaries, vacations. The best time to do the diet and the best time to get healthy is always now.

Does the diet plan help with vaginal infections?

The majority of vaginal infections are bacterial, so treating it as a yeast infection may not be effective—unless you're treating it systemically at the same time, which can help to balance the overall bacterial flora of the entire body. Many women have eliminated this problem successfully with a candida diet and others have found that it helped improve symptoms but did not get rid of them completely.

One difficulty with this part of the body is that a woman's immune-system response is regulated so that it doesn't interfere with her ability to get pregnant. That same regulation can favor the spread of candida and other infections. Therefore, trying to treat only the vaginal tissues won't work as successfully as treating the whole body.

Also, the vaginal tissue is normally acidic and the normal presence of good bacteria helps maintain the acidity. When the good bacteria are destroyed by antibiotics, it allows the pH to change and become more alkaline and other bacterial species to become dominant.

You'll obtain the best results by treating this tissue systemically and locally. Helpful ideas include inserting two acidophilus capsules twice a day into the vaginal tissue. Some women have also used boric acid suppositories to help increase the acidity.

Repeated courses of antibiotics can cause a lot of disruption of normal healthy tissue, so it may take a while to bring everything back into balance. It's not just a vaginal issue, it's a systemic issue.

Superfoods

Many of the scientific food studies concerning what people should eat should be taken with a grain of salt, as they can be based on a manufacturer's need to sell product. This research can also be influenced by who is funding the study and what they hope to gain from a positive outcome. However, the overwhelming evidence of research points to the benefits of eating specific whole foods for optimal health and well-being. This appendix includes a variety of superfoods that will help you sustain a balanced internal ecology, a strong digestive system, and ultimately, a long and healthy life.

Broccoli

From fighting cancer to cardiovascular disease, depression, diabetes, osteoporosis, high blood pressure, and aging, broccoli's health benefits are growing by the year. It is filled with vitamins A, B, and C, as well as minerals, folates, nutritious fibers, and antioxidants. For those people concerned about not getting enough vitamin C without oranges, broccoli has higher vitamin C content, as well as more calcium than a glass of milk. Broccoli is a cruciferous vegetable along with cauliflower, Brussels sprouts, cabbage, and kale. All of these are encouraged as part of any anticancer protocol, which makes them an excellent choice for everyone as a preventive measure. Cruciferous vegetables can lower thyroid hormone production, so their consumption might need to be monitored in people with thyroid issues.

Berries

Loaded with vitamins, antioxidants, colorful anthocyanins, and phytochemicals, blackberries, blueberries, cranberries, strawberries, and raspberries are the veteran superfoods. The reigning new kids on the block include acai, noni, goji, and maqui berries. Juneberries, gooseberries, lingonberries, and aronia berries are also good. Each of these berries contains an abundance of antioxidants and nutrients that have shown effectiveness against cancer, Alzheimer's disease, Parkinson's disease, diabetes, cardiovascular disease, weight gain, and high cholesterol. They contain phytochemicals that may number in the thousands. Berries don't typically provide the sugar spike found with other fruits and can often be included in small amounts when sugar problems are an issue. Each person's response in this area will vary.

Sweet Potatoes and Yams

These two vegetables are nutrient-dense and a good source of nutrients and fuel for the body when following a candida diet. Although similar in appearance and taste, they differ in other key areas. Sweet potatoes are higher in vitamin A and E, as well as iron and calcium. Yams are higher in the beneficial omega-3 oils, which might be a surprising nutrient to find in either one, since most people associate omega-3 oils with fish. Both are low on the glycemic index, which makes them a good choice for a candida diet. Aside from a nice mineral content, they also provide benefits from their carotenoid content.

ALERT

Women who eat yams do not need to worry about them affecting hormones or digestion. Those are effects created from the extracts of two plants, the Wild Mexican yam and the Chinese yam, which are completely different from yams and sweet potatoes.

Sweet potatoes are especially anti-inflammatory, making them a better choice over yams on a candida diet plan, although both have been known to work very well with this type of diet. Neither one is related to the common potato, which is associated with creating blood sugar imbalances, and therefore can be pro-inflammatory.

Tomatoes

Tomatoes make a lot of people's lists as a superfood. Known to fight cancers and heart disease, tomatoes contain a high amount of the phytochemical/carotenoid, lycopene, which has a strong antioxidant function against prostate and breast cancers. Its high nutrient content has earned the tomato the name "Red Gold," which fits well with the saying that "Health is wealth."

Avocados

Avocados are an excellent choice for adding raw fats to the diet. They are loaded with nutrients and taste great. They go well with salads, meals, and in smoothies. Like most superfoods, avocados have a mighty impact against cancer, diabetes, and heart, brain, and eye diseases. Avocados provide a lot of energy support for people on a candida diet. With more than eighty varieties to choose from, you'll have plenty of opportunity to find the one that suits your tastes. Make a guacamole spread and dip your rice cake in it, or place some sliced avocado on top. Eat them by themselves and often. The healthy fats they contain are burned up rapidly in the body. Many people find that eating several a day keeps them going and helps balance blood sugar.

Asparagus

Asparagus is a tasty superfood that can help alkalize the body, especially the urinary tract. Asparagus is another food designed by nature to help people tackle cancer, diabetes, heart disease, inflammation, and alcoholism. Anything that reduces inflammation helps to inhibit fungal candida. It's rich in nutrients like folates, antioxidants, minerals, fiber, and vitamins A, B, C, and K. Asparagus can also be a rich source of food for the intestinal bacteria, making it an excellent food for helping to create better intestinal health.

ESSENTIAL

Although some people have consumed asparagus for centuries, believing it to be an aphrodisiac, eating asparagus does not increase one's libido, stimulate milk production, or balance hormones. These effects are associated with another type of plant known as *Asparagus racemosus,* used primarily in Ayurvedic medicine.

Anyone with a bladder or urinary tract infection can usually benefit by taking herbs, supplements, and substances like grapefruit seed extract with asparagus to direct those products more specifically through the urinary system. You can tell this is happening by the smell of the asparagus sulfur compounds that are released in the urine.

Eggs

Eggs are a nutritious powerhouse packed with high-quality protein, fats, antioxidants, minerals, and vitamins. Eggs help to address heart, eye, and brain health; obesity; cancer; and diabetes. Eggs aren't just a breakfast food. Hard-boiled eggs make for a good quick snack on a candida diet. They contain amino acids needed for tissue repair and thousands of functions throughout the body. The egg yolk is especially beneficial as its high-quality fats also contain carotenoids and choline. Since choline is necessary for a baby's brain development, eggs are an important addition to the diet during pregnancy. No matter how you like to prepare them, make sure that you consider including them in your diet.

Salmon

Salmon is mostly known for its heart-health benefits due to the popularization of its omega-3 oil content. Omega-3s are also important for combating arthritis, hypertension, pregnancy, and inflammatory conditions such as cancer and multiple sclerosis. Salmon also contains vitamins A, B, and D, as well as minerals, and is a good source of protein. Concerns about mercury in fish make some people hesitant to eat fish. This hesitation may not be necessary; fish contains selenium, and selenium binds to mercury in such a tight fashion that it renders it harmless to humans. Salmon is not typically associated with high levels of mercury and is a good fish to eat, along with tilapia.

Wild-caught salmon is generally recommended over farm-raised salmon. Farm-raised salmon can contain high levels of antibiotics; it is best to avoid eating it or to limit its consumption. On this plan, it won't have much effect, but over longer periods of consumption, the antibiotics can affect the balance of good bacteria in the body. Avoid overcooking salmon to preserve the quality of the omega-3s. Salmon is a good choice for ceviche recipes and sushi.

Spices for Life

Most spices or herbs, like the plants they come from, have antifungal properties and work very well with a candida diet plan. All spices have additional effects and benefits beyond the wonderful flavors that they impart to foods. In addition to being good antifungals, some spices have antibacterial and antiparasitic properties. As representatives of Mother Nature, they all work safely and naturally to defeat infections. Used with the whole foods found on this diet, spices can potentially be life-saving.

QUESTION

What's the difference between a spice and an herb?
These terms are used interchangeably, so depending on who's speaking, it may have the same meaning. In the kitchen, an herb generally refers to the leafy part of plants, and a spice refers to the seeds, stems, roots, and flowers. In herbal formulas, the word *spice* is never used, regardless of what part of the plant is used.

Some of the spices and herbs presented here have amazing properties backed by years of scientific research. Do you have cancer or does it run in your family? Some spices have been found to block all known cancer pathways. No medication can make that claim or even come close. What about the chronic inflammation associated with most diseases? Some spices have been found to help consistently reduce inflammation. Spices and herbs can shape the expression of our genes. While exposure to toxins can activate disease genes, spices and herbs can turn those genes off. So whether it's cancer, Parkinson's, Alzheimer's, diabetes, arthritis, or a host of other conditions, or just a desire to stay healthy, it's time to spice up your life. A good spice grinder, or mortar and pestle, can help in the preparation of spices in the kitchen. Let's look at some of the powerful players in the field of spices.

Allspice

Although it smells like several other spices, allspice is one spice. Allspice oil was tested against seventy-five strains of candida and was effective against all of them. Many home remedies for foot fungus include allspice. While the spice may not be as effective as the oil, the active ingredient eugenol is present in both. Allspice has many other properties, which has helped earn its nickname All-Around Healer. It acts an anti-inflammatory, analgesic, anti-infectious, and anesthetic spice. It has been used to balance hormones and may help in managing menopause. It's good with meats and vegetables, and goes well with some other superspices like garlic, ginger, and turmeric. Anyone with digestive imbalances should consider using allspice to soothe discomfort.

Anise

Anise has demonstrated antifungal activity against several strains of candida, as well as pathogenic strains of bacteria. Anise is perfect for a candida diet and whenever digestive upset is present. Colic, constipation, ulcers, gas, and bad breath all improve with anise. It's a natural relaxant for the body. Its sweetness is used to make desserts and alcoholic beverages. Its memorable licorice flavor can enhance many dishes and goes well with allspice, cinnamon, cloves, cumin, and coriander. Stacking up on herbs in cooking is a good way to enhance and magnify their overall healing effects.

Basil

Basil is more commonly known, but many people don't realize that basil is a superspice that works well with many superfoods. It has shown effectiveness against cancer, diabetes, aging, ulcers, gout, stress, and heart disease. Since candida is associated with many of these conditions, the use of basil is a welcome addition. Some studies have also shown antifungal activity with basil.

ALERT

Basil is also available as a supplement. In this concentrated form, it can affect fertility in men and women and is not recommended during pregnancy. Take only recommended dosages or just stick to the original herb to ensure no unwanted effects.

Basil is added to many dishes worldwide. It is even used as a tea and in wedding ceremonies. It combines well with other powerful antifungal spices such as black pepper, rosemary, thyme, garlic, lemongrass, oregano, and ginger. Don't miss out on the daily health benefits that basil can provide.

Black Cumin Seed

Black cumin seed is considered a cure-all for many conditions. Its stellar reputation is believed to be due to a substance not found in other plants, thymoquinone. It helps boost and strengthen the immune system, protects against heart disease, and fights cancer. Asthma, allergies, diabetes, ulcers, and cancers are other conditions helped by black cumin seed.

With more than 160 studies on its miraculous benefits, including activity against candida, the only thing missing with this superspice is a cape. Unknown to most Americans, King Tut considered this spice important enough to be included in his tomb for travels in the afterlife. Combining it with turmeric, ginger, clove, cardamom, and cinnamon is as close to a guarantee of immortality that you'll find. Use this spice with brown rice, potatoes, lamb, and veggies. Look for it by its scientific name, *Nigella sativa*, to make sure that you're getting the real thing.

Black Pepper

This common, mild-mannered tabletop spice has an alter ego as the King of Spices. Once valued more highly than gold and traded as currency, black pepper has a royal spice pedigree and scientific studies to support its use in fighting cancer, heart disease, arthritis, Alzheimer's, vitiligo (loss of pigment in skin), hyperthyroidism, infection, digestion, obesity, and food preservation. Many supplements contain black pepper because it helps to increase absorption. Black pepper can also help stimulate production of hydrochloric acid in the stomach, which is typically lower in people with fungal candida. Research shows its effectiveness against several strains of candida, as well as against superbugs like *E. coli* and *Staph* infections. Black pepper goes well with most dishes, especially meats, soups, eggs, veggies, and salads. It combines well with many herbs and can enhance their effectiveness.

Cinnamon

This spice has an unmistakable smell that most everyone can quickly recognize. Although known for its ability to defeat diabetes and manage blood sugar levels, cinnamon has also been found to be useful against cancer, HIV, multiple sclerosis, polycystic ovarian syndrome, high cholesterol, colds, arthritis, and infections, including fungal candida.

FACT

Spices like cinnamon, cloves, black pepper, and nutmeg were so valuable that countries fought many wars in an attempt to control their trade and profits. Fought between 1500–1700, these battles were known as the Spice Wars. Many lives and ships were lost to secure profits that could sometimes be as much as 1,000 percent higher than the original price.

Cinnamon imparts a sweet flavor to dishes and goes well with allspice, cloves, ginger, cardamom, coriander, and turmeric. On a candida diet, cinnamon can help to compensate for some of the sweet taste that people may miss.

Cloves

Anyone who has experienced dental pain's searing intensity appreciates the immediate effectiveness of clove oil's numbing properties. Along with its magnificent ability to stop pain, cloves are anti-inflammatory and according to researchers in Portugal, it possesses "considerable antifungal activity" against candida. It is also effective against cancer, ulcers, hepatitis, herpes, and even mosquitoes shouldn't be forgotten. Cloves pair well with allspice, cinnamon, nutmeg, cardamom, coriander, cumin, ginger, and turmeric.

Coriander

Coriander is more commonly known as the leafy herb cilantro, but the seeds from the same plant have been used as a spice for thousands of years. Coriander is used to combat diabetes, inflammation, high cholesterol, psoriasis, and a host of digestive imbalances that include colon cancer, ulcers, inflammatory bowel and liver diseases, stomach upset, indigestion, gas, and bloating. It has been shown to inhibit fungal candida and other problematic microbes. Coriander is an excellent spice to add to a candida diet plan. It goes well with allspice, cardamom, cumin, cloves, ginger, and turmeric.

Garlic

Like cinnamon, garlic has a very distinctive smell that's easy to recognize. Unlike cinnamon, the smell isn't as pleasant. Garlic is a heavyweight in the spice world and is associated with healing properties for many illnesses and diseases. It's not an empty boast either, as there are more than 3,000 studies on garlic's benefits, including its antifungal effect. Stronger still is its antibacterial effect; it was once called Russian Penicillin. Garlic has been used to repel mosquitoes, and it is well known for its ability to improve many areas of heart health, and diabetes, and to prevent cancer. Garlic's odor is so strong that you can smell it in the skin of those who eat it. This migration to the skin also has an antiaging effect.

ESSENTIAL

Garlic is a major spice in many cultures and is a component of hundreds to thousands of dishes, and that's just the Italians. It goes well with most spices, but mixing it with coriander, cumin, lemongrass, oregano, rosemary, and thyme can produce a major antifungal punch.

Ginger

Ginger is another excellent spice to quiet the intestinal imbalances that commonly accompany candida's presence, but don't forget about its effectiveness against migraines, cancer, arthritis, asthma, heart disease, and high cholesterol. Its use has been prized in Chinese medicine for centuries. Ginger's warming effect is a great addition to many meals and drinks. It goes with allspice, cinnamon, cloves, coriander, cumin, garlic, mustard, and turmeric.

Mustard Seed

From lowly seed to King of the Condiments, mustard seeds have earned their place in history as an example of what even the tiniest seed can become. Its dense composition of antioxidants and phytonutrients makes this spice a good bet against cancer, heart disease, diabetes, arthritis, swollen prostate, migraines, and inflammation. The use of this spice has faded in and out of popularity over the past 5,000 years, but overall it has remained a top choice. Mustard is a cruciferous vegetable, like broccoli, cauliflower, cabbage, Brussels sprouts, and kale, so it may have an impact on the thyroid if consumed excessively, although this hasn't been commonly reported. Used with spices like allspice, cardamom, cinnamon, cloves, cumin, ginger, and garlic, it can enhance a multitude of flavors and benefits. Researchers from India have found that mustard seed was able to inhibit candida in the lab.

Oregano

According to mythology, oregano can create good luck, eliminate sadness, repel serpents, and help you discover your next spouse. When it's not being used in these pursuits, it can also come in handy for digestive imbalances and help eliminate parasites, pathogenic bacteria, and candida. Studies show its effectiveness against cancer, obesity, heart disease, colitis, food poisoning, insulin resistance, hypertension, and inflammation of many types. In cooking, it has a strong association with Italian foods, especially pizzas. It is a common spice in most kitchens and goes well with many dishes. Oregano is commonly paired with thyme, garlic, rosemary, and basil. It is a rich source of antioxidants and minerals. The oil form is commonly available as a supplement to help fight off candida and parasites. It is very potent in this form and only small quantities can be used at a time.

Rosemary

If you find that you're not able to remember all of the amazing properties of spices and herbs, it may be that you're in need of rosemary. Taking rosemary regularly can aid memory and help prevent cancer, diabetes, arthritis, ulcers, stress, stroke, skin rashes, liver damage, and depression. Rosemary can come in handy with excessive amounts of radiation, gamma and ultraviolet. Researchers from China found that rosemary had "significant antimicrobial effects" against candida, as well as against *Staph* infections and *E. coli*. Combining rosemary with other spice oils like clove, lemongrass, oregano, and cinnamon will further enhance its antifungal effects.

Rosemary is excellent with meats and vegetables alike. It works well in combination with oregano, sage, thyme, basil, nutmeg, cinnamon, and clove.

Turmeric

Turmeric is perhaps one of the best exports to ever come out of India. Known as Indian Gold for its bright yellow color, it is a staple not only in every household, but in most every Indian dish as well. The active ingredient, curcumin, is the main reason behind its curative properties. It has been shown to be effective against all known cancer pathways. Turmeric can both prevent cancer and cure it.

Better than aspirin for inflammation and equal to or better than chemo-therapy, without all the side effects, curcumin is the wonder herb of the day. It has proven effective against Alzheimer's, arthritis, stroke, heart disease, diabetes, cystic fibrosis, depression, and eye and gall bladder diseases. Researchers from Brazil and India have demonstrated the effectiveness of curcumin against candida. Add turmeric to eggs, salads, stews, soups, veggies, and meat dishes. Combine it with other powerful spices such as allspice, black pepper, cardamom, cumin, ginger, garlic, and coriander to create flavorful healing recipes for the whole family.

There are many other wonderful, highly effective spices and herbs not covered here. Use a wide variety of them when preparing meals to benefit from these powerhouses of nature. Make it a practice to try and use four or more spices with each meal. If you're not sure which ones work together best, you can also purchase wonderful spice combos. Chinese five-spice, curry spice, and baharat, a Middle Eastern spice combination, all make combining spices an easier task.

Spices can no longer be considered as just a way to enhance the taste of foods. Science has shown that they can be powerful aids in healing and maintaining the health of the body on a daily basis.

Standard U.S./Metric Measurement Conversions

VOLUME CONVERSIONS

U.S. Volume Measure	Metric Equivalent
⅛ teaspoon	0.5 milliliter
¼ teaspoon	1 milliliter
½ teaspoon	2 milliliters
1 teaspoon	5 milliliters
½ tablespoon	7 milliliters
1 tablespoon (3 teaspoons)	15 milliliters
2 tablespoons (1 fluid ounce)	30 milliliters
¼ cup (4 tablespoons)	60 milliliters
⅓ cup	90 milliliters
½ cup (4 fluid ounces)	125 milliliters
⅔ cup	160 milliliters
¾ cup (6 fluid ounces)	180 milliliters
1 cup (16 tablespoons)	250 milliliters
1 pint (2 cups)	500 milliliters
1 quart (4 cups)	1 liter (about)

WEIGHT CONVERSIONS

U.S. Weight Measure	Metric Equivalent
½ ounce	15 grams
1 ounce	30 grams
2 ounces	60 grams
3 ounces	85 grams
¼ pound (4 ounces)	115 grams
½ pound (8 ounces)	225 grams
¾ pound (12 ounces)	340 grams
1 pound (16 ounces)	454 grams

OVEN TEMPERATURE CONVERSIONS

Degrees Fahrenheit	Degrees Celsius
200 degrees F	95 degrees C
250 degrees F	120 degrees C
275 degrees F	135 degrees C
300 degrees F	150 degrees C
325 degrees F	160 degrees C
350 degrees F	180 degrees C
375 degrees F	190 degrees C
400 degrees F	205 degrees C
425 degrees F	220 degrees C
450 degrees F	230 degrees C

BAKING PAN SIZES

U.S.	Metric
8 × 1½ inch round baking pan	20 × 4 cm cake tin
9 × 1½ inch round baking pan	23 × 3.5 cm cake tin
11 × 7 × 1½ inch baking pan	28 × 18 × 4 cm baking tin
13 × 9 × 2 inch baking pan	30 × 20 × 5 cm baking tin
2 quart rectangular baking dish	30 × 20 × 3 cm baking tin
15 × 10 × 2 inch baking pan	30 × 25 × 2 cm baking tin (Swiss roll tin)
9 inch pie plate	22 × 4 or 23 × 4 cm pie plate
7 or 8 inch springform pan	18 or 20 cm springform or loose-bottom cake tin
9 × 5 × 3 inch loaf pan	23 × 13 × 7 cm or 2 lb narrow loaf or pâté tin
1½ quart casserole	1.5 liter casserole
2 quart casserole	2 liter casserole

Index

Note: Page numbers in **bold** indicate recipe category lists.

Acid reflux, 76–77

AIDS, candida and, 14, 27, 42, 47

Ajwain seeds, 267

Allergies, food, 97

Allspice, 286

Aminos, liquid (Bragg), 111

Amphotericin B, 46

Anise, 286

Antacids
  nutrient losses and, 78–79
  risks of, 78–79, 82–83, 84
  types of, 82
  warnings on, 79

Antibiotics
  benefits of, 24
  causing fungal candida, 14
  creating antibiotic-resistant bacteria, 29–30
  double-edged sword of, 14
  downsides of, 10, 12–13, 17–18, 22–24
  hidden epidemic of, 22–24
  how they affect system, 17–18
  mandate to protect from, 19
  methods enabling candida transformation, 23–24
  myth of, 24–25
  never taken, yet having candida, 15
  paradox of, 22
  probiotics offsetting effects of. *See* Probiotics
  reducing gut biodiversity, 17–18
  relating health issues to, 18
  triggering fungal conversion, 12–13

Antibodies, blood tests for, 37–38

Antifungals, 94

Anytime Lemon-Basil Water, 266

Appetizers, **121**–31
  Applesauce, 122
  Avocado with Grapefruit and Sweet Onion Salsa, 130
  Baba Ghanoush, 129
  Cinnamon–Spiced Applesauce, 123
  Cucumber Relish, 129
  Guacamole Picado, 131
  Mango Fruit Salad, 125
  Miguel's Guacamole, 126
  Pink Applesauce, 122
  Salvadoran Guacamole, 126
  Spiced Tropical Fruit, 124
  Spicy Guacamole, 127
  Tomato and Jicama Guacamole, 128

Apples
  about: applesauce as sweetener, 122
  Applesauce, 122
  Cinnamon–Spiced Applesauce, 123
  Pink Applesauce, 122

Arroz con Pollo (Rice with Chicken), 211

Artichokes and potatoes, roasted, 202

Asparagus
  about: benefits of, 284; as superfood, 284
  Blanched Asparagus or String Beans, 185

Chicken Soup with Asparagus, 172

Roasted Asparagus, 199

Avocados
  about: benefits of, 116, 283; on huevos rancheros, 116; as superfood, 283
  Avocado with Grapefruit and Sweet Onion Salsa, 130
  Avocado-Zucchini Soup, 169
  Guacamole Picado, 131
  Guacamole Soup, 168
  Miguel's Guacamole, 126
  Salvadoran Guacamole, 126
  Spiced Crab and Avocado Salad, 152
  Spicy Guacamole, 127
  Tomato and Jicama Guacamole, 128
  Tuna and Avocado Spread, 153

Azoles, 46–47

Baba Ghanoush, 129

Baby Red Potatoes with Cilantro, 208

Bacillus subtilis, 63

Baked Brown Rice, 212

Baked Meatballs, 246

Baked Tilapia, 230

Bananas, in Spiced Tropical Fruit, 124

Barbecued Teriyaki Salmon, 232

Basil
  about: benefits of, 287
  Anytime Lemon-Basil Water, 266
  Basil and Sage Steak Sauce, 150
  Lemon and Basil Chicken, 219

Roasted Potatoes with Basil, 209
Tomato Sauce with Basil, 137
Baths, hot, 100, 102, 273–74, 276,
  277, 279
Beef, **243**
  about: candida-friendly spaghetti
    and meatballs, 246; cooking
    steak tip, 150; making good
    burgers, 159; marinating flank
    steak overnight, 149; sirloin
    steak/strip loin/strip steak, 252
  Baked Meatballs, 246
  Basil and Sage Steak Sauce, 150
  Beef (or Chicken) Skewers, 259
  Beef and Vegetable Rice, 247
  Beef Stock, 166
  Beef Tenderloin in Morita Chili
    and Tomatillo Sauce, 260
  Bowl of Red (Basic Chili), 251
  Flank Steak Marinade, 149
  Green Sun Tea Spa Water, 268
  Hamburger or Ground Turkey
    Hash, 255
  Lettuce and Beef, 158
  Lime-Cilantro Soup, 173
  Long-Simmered Beef Seasoned
    with Chile Pasilla, 262
  Marinated Beef Tenderloin, 244
  Marinated Rib Roast, 245
  Mexican Meatloaf, 261
  Mexican-Style Chili, 248
  Mishmash, 247
  Pepper Steak, 252
  The Perfect Steak, 251
  Picadillo, 249
  South American Chili, 163
  Spicy Beef Chili Without Beans,
    250
  Steak Marinade, 244
  Steak with Basil and Sage Dry
    Rub, 253
  Steak with Rosemary and
    Tomatoes, 254

Sunrise Scrambler, 120
Beet Soup, 174
Berkhout, Christine, 20
Berries
  about: benefits of, 282; as
    superfood, 282
  Mango Fruit Salad, 125
  Spiced Tropical Fruit, 124
Beverages, **265**–69
  Anytime Lemon-Basil Water, 266
  Cinnamon-Infused Coffee, 266
  Cinnamon Tea, 266
  Digest Tea, 267
  Long-Life Tea, 269
  Spa Water, 268
Bifidobacterium, 57–58
Black cumin seed, 287
Black walnut, 52
Blanca's Spicy Cauli-Rice, 189
Blenders and juicers, 108–9, 170
Blood pressure, 51, 53, 70, 94, 279,
  282
Blood sugar imbalances, candida
  and
    about: overview of, 66
  Blood Sugar Protocol for, 68–69,
    272
  diabetes and, 71–74, 100, 272
  gestational diabetes and, 72–74
  how blood sugar works and, 66
  hyperglycemia (high blood sugar)
    and, 69–71
  hypoglycemia (low blood sugar)
    and, 66–69
  insulin and, 66, 70, 71
  prediabetes (insulin resistance)
    and, 66, 69–70, 71, 72, 272
  regulating blood sugar, 68
  smoking and, 72
Blood Sugar Protocol, 68–69, 272
Blood tests
  for blood sugar, 67, 69–70
  for candida, 37–38

Book overview, 10, 18
Bowel movements, 272–73. *See also*
  Constipation
Bowl of Red (Basic Chili), 251
Bragg Liquid Aminos, 111
Braised Butternut Squash, 203
Braised Fingerling Potatoes, 206
Braised Sweet Onions, 190
Breakfast ideas, **115**–20
  Brown Rice Frittata, 118
  Egg and Spinach Bake, 118
  Egg Lasagna, 117
  Farmers' Scrambler, 119
  Green Frittata, 118
  Huevos Rancheros Without
    Tortillas, 116
  South of the Border Scrambler,
    120
  Sunrise Scrambler, 120
Breast cancer, 283
Breastfeeding and breast milk, 58,
  60, 61, 277
Broccoli
  about: benefits of, 282; as
    superfood, 282
  Green Frittata, 118
Broths and stocks, 107. *See also*
  Soups and stews
Brown rice
  about: brown rice benefits, 100; as
    pasta alternative, 143
  Another Herbed Rice, 215
  Arroz con Pollo (Rice with
    Chicken), 211
  Baked Brown Rice, 212
  Beef and Vegetable Rice, 247
  Brown Rice Frittata, 118
  Brown Rice Polenta, 213
  Brown Rice with Peas, 196
  Chicken, Onions, Tomatoes over
    Rice, 223
  Five-Spice Rice, 216
  Green Brown Rice, 211

Herbed Rice Pilaf, 214
Holiday Rice, 212
Mishmash, 247
Picadillo, 249
Pineapple, Red Pepper, and
  Brown Rice Salad, 162
Salmon with Fresh Ginger Sauce
  and Rice, 231

Cabbage
  Harvest Vegetable Stew, 176
  Pineapple Slaw, 186
Calabacitas, 187
Calabacitas Scramble, 187
Calcium, 60, 79, 81–82
Cancer, 28
  antacids and, 83
  antibiotics and, 24–25
  candida and, 13, 14, 28
  development of, 28
  herbs for, 49, 51, 53
  inflammation and, 28, 86–87, 98
  Lactobacillus and, 57, 77
  meats and, 98
  nystatin and, 47
  obesity and, 85
  vitamin B$_{12}$ and, 80–81
Candida
  antibiotics triggering. *See*
    Antibiotics
  balanced vs. unbalanced systems
    and, 12
  behavior influences, 12
  benefits of, 13
  body masking appearance of, 18
  danger of, perspective, 27–28
  diagnosing. *See* Diagnosing
    candida
  diet and, 28–29, 33–34. *See also*
    Candida diet
  doctors and, 25–27
  dual nature of, 12
  ecosystem diversity and, 17–18

everything being food for, 92–93
factors exacerbating, 28–30
first cases, 20
forms of, 20–21
as friend or foe, 13
history of, 20–21
inflammation and. *See*
  Inflammation
medications, 29. *See also*
  Antibiotics
microscopic views of, 13
other pathogens and, 29–30
pets having, 21
as polymorph, 21
research perspective, 25–27
stress and, 29
symptoms. *See* Symptoms of
  candida
triggers converting yeast to
  fungus, 12–13
two states of, 12
virulence of, 21
what it is, 12–14
who can get it, 14
from yeast to fungus, 12–13, 23
Candida, yeast form
  appearance of cells, 13
  benefits of, 13
  compared to fungal form, 12–13
Candida albicans, 20–21, 26, 77–
  78, 91, 276
Candida diet, 89–104. *See also*
  specific recipes and main
  ingredients
  about: overview of, 89
  adding foods back in week 9, 103,
    277, 278–79
  age range to do, 279
  antifungals and, 94
  basic structure of, 97
  best time to do, 279
  children and, 277
  "die-off, detoxification and, 277

epigenetics and, 95–96
essentials of, 90–95
everything being food for candida
  and, 92–93
exercise and, 274
fasting and, 278
fats and, 92
feeling worse before better on,
  277
fermented foods and, 93–94
food allergies and, 97
high cholesterol and, 276
inflammation and, 94–95
menstrual flow and, 278
nature's pharmacy/gifts and, 96,
  109–10
origins of, 90
plant benefits, 110
power of nature and, 95–96
pregnancy and, 277–78
protein and, 92
repeating, 277
SAD and, 28, 95
sugars and. *See* Sugars
support for, 109
sweating and, 100–103, 273–74,
  279
taking medications during, 274–75
time commitment, 103–4
vaginal infections and, 279–80
vegetarians/vegans and, 275
Yes Foods, 97–103, 275
Candida dubliniensis, 21
Caprylic acid, 59–60
Caribbean Chicken with Pineapple
  Salsa, 226
Carrots
  Nikki's Stew, 178
  Roasted Carrots, 198
  Roasted Carrot Soup, 198
  Vegetable Chowder, 175
  Vegetable Curry, 194
  Vegetable Stock, 167

Cauliflower
Blanca's Spicy Cauli-Rice, 189
Vegetable Curry, 194
Celiac disease, 86–87
Chemicals
babies born with, 101
body absorbing, binding to fat,
100–101
increasing inflammation, 101–2
negative effects of, 100–102
stimulating response favorable to
candida, 101
sweating out. See Sweating
volume in environment, 101
Chesapeake Stew, 235
Chicken, **217**–26
about: cooking, 218; factual
tidbit about, 224; safety when
cooking, 160; sage with, 219
Arroz con Pollo (Rice with
Chicken), 211
Beef (or Chicken) Skewers, 259
Caribbean Chicken with
Pineapple Salsa, 226
Chicken, Onions, Tomatoes over
Rice, 223
Chicken Cacciatore with Porcini
Mushrooms, 225
Chicken Pizzaiola, 224
Chicken Soup with Asparagus,
172
Chicken Stock, 166
Chunky Chicken Salad, 160
Lemon and Basil Chicken, 219
Marinated Chicken, 218
Roasted Chicken with Oregano,
220
Summer Chicken Salad, 184
Tarragon-Lemon Chicken, 222
Tuscan Chicken, 221
Children, candida diet and, 277
Children, sweating and, 277
Chlorine, 63

Cholesterol, 47, 57, 100, 276, 282,
288, 289, 290
Cilantro
Baby Red Potatoes with Cilantro,
208
Green Brown Rice, 211
Lime-Cilantro Soup, 173
Cinnamon, 53–54, 288
Cinnamon-Infused Coffee, 266
Cinnamon–Spiced Applesauce, 123
Cinnamon Tea, 266
Citrus
about: candida diet and, 99;
mucus levels and, 99
Anytime Lemon-Basil Water, 266
Avocado with Grapefruit and
Sweet Onion Salsa, 130
Lemon and Basil Chicken, 219
Lemon-Basil Green Beans, 186
Lime-Cilantro Soup, 173
Spa Water, 268
Tarragon-Lemon Chicken, 222
Clostridium difficile, 30, 82
Cloves, 54–55, 289
Coffee, cinnamon-infused, 266
Colloidal silver, 61–62
Constipation, 80, 84–85. *See also*
Bowel movements
Cooking, 105–13. *See also specific
recipes and main ingredients*
about: overview of, 105
dining out instead of, 111–12
GMOs and, 112–13
keeping it simple, 110–11
microwaving effects and, 111
preparation importance, 106
time requirements, 106
Cordero en Chilindron (Lamb in
Chilindron Sauce), 256
Coriander, 289
Corn
Chesapeake Stew, 235
Corn Soup, 179

Lime-Cilantro Soup, 173
Mixed Vegetables, 188
Roasted Corn Soup, 201
Roasted Corn with Herbs, 201
Spicy Beef Chili Without Beans,
250
Crook, Dr. William, 10
Cucumbers
Cucumber Relish, 129
Gazpacho, 170
Red and Green Gazpacho, 183
Spa Water, 268
Cumin seed, black, 287
Curried vegetables, 194

Diabetes, 71–74, 100, 272
Diagnosing candida, 31–43. *See
also* Symptoms of candida
about: overview of, 31
antifungal diet for, 33–34
constipation, 80
factors considered, 32–34
health history and, 32
tests for. *See* Testing for candida
Diet. *See also* Candida diet
candida and, 28–29
diagnosing candida and, 33–34
Diflucan. *See* Azoles
Digestive problems, 75–87. *See also*
Antacids; Hydrochloric acid (HCl);
Ulcers
acid reflux, 76–77
bacterial flora and, 77
bowel movements and, 272–73
constipation, 84–85
folic acid (vitamin B$_9$) and, 81
gastritis, 77–78
gluten intolerance, 86–87
iodine and, 80
iron and, 79–80
low HCl levels, 76, 83–84
minerals and, 81–82
nutrient losses and, 78–79

obesity and, 85
protein and, 79
testing for HCl and, 83
vitamin B$_{12}$ and, 80–81
Digest Tea, 267
Dining out, 111–12
Doctors, candida and, 25–27

Echinocandins, 48
E. coli, candida and, 29
Eggplants
Baba Ghanoush, 129
Ratatouille, 193
Slow-Cooker Mediterranean Stew
(or Lamb Mediterranean Stew),
177
Eggs
about: benefits of, 99–100, 284;
cholesterol concerns answered,
100; as superfood, 284
Brown Rice Frittata, 118
Calabacitas Scramble, 187
Egg and Spinach Bake, 118
Egg Lasagna, 117
Egg Salad, 153
Farmers' Scrambler, 119
Green Frittata, 118
Huevos Rancheros Without
Tortillas, 116
Niçoise Salad, 161
Salvadoran Guacamole, 126
South of the Border Scrambler, 120
Sunrise Scrambler, 120
Epigenetics, 95–96
Exercise, 274

FAQ, 271–80
Farmers' Scrambler, 119
Fasting, 278
Fats, 92
Fatty acids, 59–61
about: treating candida with, 59
caprylic acid, 59–60

lauric acid, 61
undecenoic acid, 20, 60–61
Fecal transplant, 56
Feedback loops, 33
Fennel, treating candida with, 55
Fermented foods, 93–94
Fish and seafood, **227–41**
about: as brain food, 231; cooking
shrimp, 239; salmon benefits,
231, 285; as superfood, 285;
tuna dish varieties, 236
Baked Tilapia, 230
Barbecued Teriyaki Salmon, 232
Chesapeake Stew, 235
Fish Ceviche, 238
Grilled Fish with Salsa Fresca,
237
Grilled Mahi-Mahi, 233
Grilled Tiger Shrimp with Two
Sauces, 239
Mahi-Mahi with Creole Sauce, 229
Marinated Fish, 228
Maryellen's Tuna Salad, 154
Mexican Fish, 234
Niçoise Salad, 161
Red and Green Gazpacho, 183
Salmon with Fresh Ginger Sauce
and Rice, 231
Salsa Tuna, 236
Scallops á la Adam, 230
Seafood Soup, 240–41
Spiced Crab and Avocado Salad,
152
Tuna and Avocado Spread, 153
Tuna Salad Roll-Up, 159
Tuna Salad with Beefsteak
Tomatoes, 156
Fit Fries, 205
Five-Spice Rice, 216
Flank Steak Marinade, 149
Food allergies, 97
French fries, oven-baked, 204
Fries, baked, 204, 205

Fruits. See also specific fruits
about: avoiding during candida
diet, 98; candida-fighting
benefits, 99, 110; epigenetic
behavior and, 95–96; GMOs,
112–13; on kebabs, 125
Spiced Tropical Fruit, 124
Fuller, Rachel, 90

Garlic, 49–50, 289–90
Gas chromatography, 36
Gastritis, 77–78
Genetically modified organisms
(GMOs), 112–13
GERD (Gastro-Esophageal Reflux
Disease), 77
Gestational diabetes, 72–74
Ginger
about: benefits of, 290; dipping
sauce, 144
Ginger Sauce, 144
Gluten intolerance, 86–87
GMOs, 112–13
Grapefruit. See Citrus
Grapefruit seed extract, 50–51
Grated Potato Pancakes, 210
Green beans
Chesapeake Stew, 235
Harvest Vegetable Stew, 176
Lemon-Basil Green Beans, 186
Niçoise Salad, 161
Green Brown Rice, 211
Green Frittata, 118
Green Herb Sauce/Marinade, 145
Grilled Fish with Salsa Fresca, 237
Grilled Mahi-Mahi, 233
Grilled Portobello with Chipotle
Sauce, 263
Grilled Tiger Shrimp with Two
Sauces, 239
Grocery list, 107–8
Guacamole, 126
Guacamole Picado, 131

Guacamole Soup, 168
Salvadoran Guacamole, 126
Spicy Guacamole, 127
Tomato and Jicama Guacamole, 128

Hamburger or Ground Turkey Hash, 255
Harvest Vegetable Stew, 176
Hash, hamburger or ground turkey, 255
Hazen, Elizabeth Lee, 90
Health history, 32
Helicobacter pylori (h. pylori), 77
Herbed rice dishes, 214, 215
Herbs and spices, 49–56, 285–92
    about: difference between, 285; effectiveness in treating candida, 94, 96, 285–86; general benefits of, 285–86; researching on Internet, 55–56; tradition and value of, 49
    allspice, 286
    anise, 286
    basil, 287
    black cumin seed, 287
    black pepper, 288
    black walnut, 52
    cinnamon, 53–54, 288
    cloves, 54–55, 289
    coriander, 289
    fennel, 55
    garlic, 49–50, 289–90
    ginger, 290
    grapefruit seed extract, 50–51
    mustard seed, 290
    olive leaf extract, 51–52
    oregano, 50, 291
    other herbs, 55–56
    pau d'arco, 51
    rosemary, 53, 291
    tea tree oil, 52–53
    thyme, 54

turmeric, 291–92
Histamine, 57, 93, 94–95, 98, 99
History of candida, 20–21
Holiday Rice, 212
Hot Sauce, 140
Huevos Rancheros Without Tortillas, 116
Hugo's Emerald Mayonnaise, 147
Hwp1 (Hyphal wall protein), 86
Hydrating, 102–3, 276
Hydrochloric acid (HCl). *See also* Antacids; Ulcers
    acid reflux and, 76–77
    constipation and, 84–85
    digesting meats and, 80
    folic acid (vitamin B_9) and, 81
    gastritis and, 77–78
    iodine and, 80
    iron and, 79–80
    low levels of, 76, 83–84
    nutrient losses and, 78–79
    protein and, 79
    testing for, 83
    treating high levels naturally, 78
    treating low levels, 83–84
    vitamin B_{12} and, 80–81
Hyperglycemia (high blood sugar), 69–71
Hypoglycemia (low blood sugar), 66–69

Immune system
    antibiotics suppressing, 23, 24
    cancer and, 28
    controlling candida, 21
    determining strength of, 27
    factors exacerbating candida, 28–30
    inflammation and, 15–16. *See also* Inflammation
    non-suppressed, candida and, 14
    polymorph nature of candida and, 21

research perspective on candida and, 25–26
    suppressed, dangers of, 27–28
    virulence of candida and, 21
    weakened/suppressed, triggering candida fungus, 12–13
Immunoglobulins, blood tests for, 37–38
Immunosuppressive drugs, candida and, 25, 27–28, 58
Inflammation, 15–16
    cancer and, 28, 86–87, 98
    candida diet and, 94–95
    candida promoting, 93
    candida thriving on, 18
    chemicals (mercury) increasing, 101–2
    conditions associated with candida and, 16–17
    constipation and, 85
    fermented foods and, 93–94
    gluten intolerance and, 86–87
    immune system and, 15–16
    influencing all diseases, 18
    linking candida to multiple conditions/symptoms, 15
    stool tests and, 36–37
Ingredients. *See specific main ingredients*
Insulin resistance. *See* Prediabetes (insulin resistance)
Iodine, 80
Iron, 79–80

Jalapeño Blender Mayonnaise, 148
Jicama, in Tomato and Jicama Guacamole, 128
Juicers and blenders, 108–9
Juicing, 108–9

Kebabs/skewers
    about: history of, 258
    Beef (or Chicken) Skewers, 259

Fruit Kebabs, 125
Hot and Creamy Skewer Dip, 259
Lamb Kebabs, 258
Ketchup, homemade, 204
Kiwis, in Spiced Tropical Fruit, 124

Lactobacillus , 57, 77
Lactose intolerance, 57
Lamb
    Cordero en Chilindron (Lamb in
        Chilindron Sauce), 256
    Lamb Kebabs, 258
    Lamb Mediterranean Stew, 177
    Mustard-Glazed Lamb, 257
Lapacho (pau d'arco), 51
Lasagna, egg, 117
Lauric acid, 61
Leeks, in Potato-Leek Soup, 171
Lettuce and Beef, 158
Long-Life Tea, 269
Long-Simmered Beef Seasoned with
    Chile Pasilla, 262
Lufenuron, 62–63
Lunch, 157–63
    Chunky Chicken Salad, 160
    Lettuce and Beef, 158
    Niçoise Salad, 161
    Pineapple, Red Pepper, and
        Brown Rice Salad, 162
    South American Chili, 163
    Tuna Salad Roll-Up, 159
Lupus, 15, 24

Magnesium, 60, 79, 81–82
Mahi-mahi. See Fish and seafood
Mangoes
    Mango Fruit Salad, 125
    Mango Pico de Gallo, 136
    Spiced Tropical Fruit, 124
Marinades. See Sauces and
    marinades
Marinara Sauce, 138
Marinated Beef Tenderloin, 244

Marinated Chicken, 218
Marinated Fish, 228
Marinated Rib Roast, 245
Maryellen's Tuna Salad, 154
Mayonnaise
    Homemade Mayonnaise, 146
    Hugo's Emerald Mayonnaise, 147
    Jalapeño Blender Mayonnaise,
        148
    Roasted Bell Pepper Mayonnaise,
        146
Measurement conversions, 293
Meats, candida and, 97–98. See
    also specific meats
Medications. See also Antacids
    for candida. See Medications, for
        candida
    promoting candida, 29. See also
        Antibiotics
    side effects of, 48
    taking during candida diet,
        274–75
    test requirement for prescribing, 69
    for ulcers, 82–83
Medications, for candida, 46–48
    amphotericin B, 46
    antifungal resistance to, 48
    azoles, 46–47
    candida diet and, 48
    echinocandins, 48
    nystatin, 47, 90
    ongoing research for, 48
Menstrual flow, 278
Metchnikoff, Élie, 56
Metric measurement conversions,
    293
Mexican Fish, 234
Mexican Meatloaf, 261
Mexican-Style Chili, 248
Microwaving, effects of, 111
Miguel's Guacamole, 126
Minerals, 81–82, 275. See also
    specific minerals

Mint
    Digest Tea, 267
    Spa Water, 268
    Tomato-Mint Sauce, 142
    Tomato-Mint Soup, 142
Mishmash, 247
Mixed Vegetables, 188
Multiple sclerosis, 15, 84, 85, 276,
    285, 288
Multistrain probiotics, 58–59
Mushrooms
    about: absorbing water, 192;
        candida and, 139; cleaning, 192
    Chicken Cacciatore with Porcini
        Mushrooms, 225
    Grilled Portobello with Chipotle
        Sauce, 263
    Porcini Sauce, 139
    Spicy Asian-Inspired Mushrooms,
        192
    Vegetable Chowder, 175
Mustard-Glazed Lamb, 257
Mustard seed, 290

Niçoise Salad, 161
Nikki's Stew, 178
Nozoral. See Azoles
Nutrient losses, 78–79
Nystatin, 47, 90

Obesity, 85
Okra
    Chesapeake Stew, 235
    Slow-Cooker Mediterranean Stew
        (or Lamb Mediterranean Stew),
        177
    Spicy Okra with Tomatoes, 191
Olive leaf extract, 51–52
Onions
    Avocado with Grapefruit and
        Sweet Onion Salsa, 130
    Braised Sweet Onions, 190
    Nikki's Stew, 178

Pico de Gallo, 136
Roasted Peppery Onions, 201
Oral Glucose Tolerance Test (OGTT), 67
Oregano, 50, 291
Oven-Baked French Fries, 204

Paleo stew, 178
Pancakes, potato, 210
Papayas, in Spiced Tropical Fruit, 124
Parasites
herbs for, 51, 52, 291
testing for, 36
Pasta alternatives, 138, 143, 246
Pau d'arco, 51
Peas
Brown Rice with Peas, 196
Five-Spice Rice, 216
South American Chili, 163
Peppers
about: adding heat with, 140; roasted bell peppers for multiple purposes, 200
Chipotle Sauce, 263
Gazpacho, 170
Jalapeño Blender Mayonnaise, 148
Pineapple, Red Pepper, and Brown Rice Salad, 162
Ratatouille, 193
Roasted Bell Pepper Mayonnaise, 146
Roasted Pepper Fillets, 200
Pepper Steak, 252
Pets, candida and, 21
Picadillo, 249
Pico de Gallo, 136
Pineapple
about: presentation using, 124
Mango Fruit Salad, 125
Pineapple, Red Pepper, and Brown Rice Salad, 162

Pineapple Salsa, 135, 226
Pineapple Slaw, 186
Spiced Tropical Fruit, 124
Pink Applesauce, 122
Polymerase chain reaction (PCR), 37
Polymorph, candida as, 21
Porcine endogenous retrovirus (PERV), 97–98, 275–76
Porcini Sauce, 139
Pork, candida and, 97–98, 275–76
Potatoes
Baby Red Potatoes with Cilantro, 208
Braised Fingerling Potatoes, 206
Farmers' Scrambler, 119
Fit Fries, 205
Grated Potato Pancakes, 210
Harvest Vegetable Stew, 176
Mixed Vegetables, 188
New Potato Salad, 207
Niçoise Salad, 161
Nikki's Stew, 178
Oven-Baked French Fries, 204
Potato-Leek Soup, 171
Roasted Artichokes and Potatoes, 202
Roasted Potatoes with Basil, 209
Vegetable Curry, 194
Prediabetes (insulin resistance), 66, 69–70, 71, 72, 272
Pregnancies, candida and, 72–74, 277–78
Probiotics, 56–59
benefits of, 56
Bifidobacterium, 57–58
defined, 56
doctors recommending, 23
fecal transplant for, 56
Lactobacillus , 57, 77
multistrain, 58–59
offsetting antibiotic effects, 23, 25
optimizing number of probiotic species, 56

regimen for taking, 103–4
stool tests and, 36, 37
streptococcus thermophilus, 58
Prostaglandins, 93
Protease enzymes, 70
Protein, 79, 92
Puttanesca Sauce, 143

Questions and answers, about candida, 271–80

Ranchero Sauce, 141
Ratatouille, 193
Recipes. See specific categories of recipes; specific main ingredients
Research perspective, on candida, 25–27
Restaurants, dining at, 111–12
Rice. See Blanca's Spicy Cauli-Rice; Brown rice
Roasted Artichokes and Potatoes, 202
Roasted Asparagus, 199
Roasted Bell Pepper Mayonnaise, 146
Roasted Carrots, 198
Roasted Carrot Soup, 198
Roasted Chicken with Oregano, 220
Roasted Corn Soup, 201
Roasted Corn with Herbs, 201
Roasted Pepper Fillets, 200
Roasted Peppery Onions, 201
Roasted Plum Tomatoes, 198
Roasted Potatoes with Basil, 209
Roasted Squash Medley, 199
Roasted Sweet Potatoes, 200
Roasted Zucchini, 199
Rosemary, 53, 291

Sage, chicken with, 219
Salads, 151–56. See also Sandwiches and wraps
Chunky Chicken Salad, 160

Egg Salad, 153

Fresh Tuna with Watercress Salad, 155

Mango Fruit Salad, 125

Maryellen's Tuna Salad, 154

New Potato Salad, 207

Niçoise Salad, 161

Pineapple, Red Pepper, and Brown Rice Salad, 162

Pineapple Slaw, 186

Spiced Crab and Avocado Salad, 152

Summer Chicken Salad, 184

Tuna and Avocado Spread, 153

Tuna Salad with Beefsteak Tomatoes, 156

Saliva tests, 39–40. See also Spit Test

Salmon. See Fish and seafood

Salsas. See Sauces and marinades

Salvadoran Guacamole, 126

Sandwiches and wraps

about: making good burgers, 159

Chunky Chicken Salad, 160

Lettuce and Beef, 158

Spiced Crab and Avocado Salad on, 152

Tuna Salad Roll-Up, 159

Sauces and marinades, **133**–50

about: canned salsa, 137; dipping salsa/sauce, 134, 144; making your own tomato sauce, 117

Avocado with Grapefruit and Sweet Onion Salsa, 130

Basil and Sage Steak Sauce, 150

Chipotle Sauce, 263

Flank Steak Marinade, 149

Ginger Sauce, 144

Green Herb Sauce/Marinade, 145

Homemade Ketchup, 204

Homemade Mayonnaise, 146

Hot and Creamy Skewer Dip, 259

Hot Sauce, 140

Hugo's Emerald Mayonnaise, 147

Jalapeño Blender Mayonnaise, 148

Mango Pico de Gallo, 136

Marinara Sauce, 138

Morita Chili and Tomatillo Sauce, 260

Pico de Gallo, 136

Pineapple Salsa, 135, 226

Porcini Sauce, 139

Puttanesca Sauce, 143

Ranchero Sauce, 141

Roasted Bell Pepper Mayonnaise, 146

Salsa Fresca, 134

Salsa Tuna, 236

Salsa Verde, 136

Simple Salsa Recipe, 120

Tomato-Mint Sauce, 142

Tomato Sauce with Basil, 137

Scallops. See Fish and seafood

Seafood. See Fish and seafood

Secreted aspartyl proteases (SAPs), 70

Shallots, crispy, spinach with, 195

Shaw, Dr. William, 39

Shrimp. See Fish and seafood

Sides, **180**–216

about: excellent for holidays, 185

Another Herbed Rice, 215

Arroz con Pollo (Rice with Chicken), 211

Baby Red Potatoes with Cilantro, 208

Baked Brown Rice, 212

Blanca's Spicy Cauli-Rice, 189

Blanched Asparagus or String Beans, 185

Braised Butternut Squash, 203

Braised Fingerling Potatoes, 206

Braised Sweet Onions, 190

Brown Rice Polenta, 213

Brown Rice with Peas, 196

Calabacitas, 187

Calabacitas Scramble, 187

Fit Fries, 205

Five-Spice Rice, 216

Grated Potato Pancakes, 210

Green Brown Rice, 211

Herbed Rice Pilaf, 214

Holiday Rice, 212

Lemon-Basil Green Beans, 186

Mixed Vegetables, 188

New Potato Salad, 207

Oven-Baked French Fries, 204

Pineapple Slaw, 186

Ratatouille, 193

Red and Green Gazpacho, 183

Roasted Artichokes and Potatoes, 202

Roasted Asparagus, 199

Roasted Carrots, 198

Roasted Corn with Herbs, 201

Roasted Pepper Fillets, 200

Roasted Peppery Onions, 201

Roasted Plum Tomatoes, 198

Roasted Potatoes with Basil, 209

Roasted Sweet Potatoes, 200

Roasted Zucchini, 199

Spiced Sweet Purée, 182

Spicy Asian-Inspired Mushrooms, 192

Spicy Okra with Tomatoes, 191

Spinach with Crispy Shallots, 195

Summer Chicken Salad, 184

Swiss Chard with Olives, 197

Vegetable Curry, 194

Silver, colloidal, 61–62

Simple Salsa Recipe, 120

Simplicity, of diet, 110–11

Skewers. See Kebabs/skewers

Slow-Cooker Mediterranean Stew (or Lamb Mediterranean Stew), 235

Slow cookers, using, 106

Smoking, 72

Snacks

applesauce as, 122
stocking, 107–8
Sorrel, in Hugo's Emerald
  Mayonnaise, 147
Soups and stews, **165**–79
  about: broths and stocks, 107;
    Paleo stew, 178; using blender
    to blend, 170
  Avocado-Zucchini Soup, 169
  Beef Stock, 166
  Beet Soup, 174
  Bowl of Red (Basic Chili), 251
  Chesapeake Stew, 235
  Chicken Soup with Asparagus,
    172
  Chicken Stock, 166
  Corn Soup, 179
  Gazpacho, 170
  Guacamole Soup, 168
  Harvest Vegetable Stew, 176
  Lamb Mediterranean Stew, 177
  Lime-Cilantro Soup, 173
  Mexican-Style Chili, 248
  Nikki's Stew, 178
  Potato-Leek Soup, 171
  Red and Green Gazpacho, 183
  Roasted Carrot Soup, 198
  Roasted Corn Soup, 201
  Seafood Soup, 240–41
  Slow-Cooker Mediterranean Stew,
    177
  South American Chili, 163
  Spicy Beef Chili Without Beans,
    250
  Tomato-Mint Soup, 142
  Vegetable Chowder, 175
  Vegetable Curry (puréed), 194
  Vegetable Stock, 167
South American Chili, 163
South of the Border Scrambler, 120
Spa Water, 268
Spiced Crab and Avocado Salad,
  152

Spiced Sweet Purée, 182
Spiced Tropical Fruit, 124
Spicy Asian-Inspired Mushrooms,
  192
Spicy Beef Chili Without Beans, 250
Spicy Guacamole, 127
Spicy Okra with Tomatoes, 191
Spinach
  Egg and Spinach Bake, 118
  Egg Lasagna, 117
  Hamburger or Ground Turkey
    Hash, 255
  Hugo's Emerald Mayonnaise, 147
  Spinach with Crispy Shallots, 195
  Vegetable Chowder, 175
Spit Test, 40–41
Sporanox. *See* Azoles
Squash
  about: spaghetti squash pasta,
    138, 246
  Avocado-Zucchini Soup, 169
  Braised Butternut Squash, 203
  Calabacitas, 187
  Nikki's Stew, 178
  Ratatouille, 193
  Roasted Squash Medley, 199
  Roasted Zucchini, 199
  Slow-Cooker Mediterranean Stew
    (or Lamb Mediterranean Stew),
    177
  Vegetable Chowder, 175
Standard American Diet SAD, 28, 95
Staphylococcus aureus, 30
Steak. *See* Beef
Stocks and broths, 107. *See also*
  Soups and stews
Stool tests, 36–37
Strawberries. *See* Berries
Streptococcus thermophilus, 58
Stress, 29
String beans, blanched, 185
Sugars, 90–92
  annual personal consumption, 91

antifungal diet and, 33–34. *See
  also* Candida diet
balanced diet and, 92
blood sugar and. *See* Blood sugar
  imbalances, candida and
candida thriving on, 28–29, 33–
  34, 38, 91
diseases and, 32
functions and functioning of,
  90–92
lactose intolerance, 57
yeasty candida fermenting,
  breaking down, 12
Summer Chicken Salad, 184
Sunrise Scrambler, 120
Superfoods, 281–92. *See also
  specific superfoods*
Supplements
  amino acid, 275
  asparagus, 284
  black walnut, 52
  to boost immune system, 103
  breastfeeding and, 277
  cinnamon, 54
  cloves, 55
  fennel, 55
  folic acid (vitamin B_9), 81
  garlic, 50
  HCl, 83–84
  iron, 80
  olive leaf extract, 52
  oregano, 50, 291
  pau d'arco, 51
  rosemary, 53
  taking during candida diet, 273
Support, for diet, 109
Sweating, 100–103, 273–74, 277, 279
Sweetener, applesauce as, 122. *See
  also* Sugars
Sweet potatoes and yams
  about: benefits of, 282–83; as
    superfood, 282
  Fit Fries, 205

Nikki's Stew, 178
Roasted Sweet Potatoes, 200
Spiced Sweet Purée, 182
Swiss chard
Chicken Soup with Asparagus, 172
Swiss Chard with Olives, 197
Symptoms of candida, 33
diagnosing candida and, 33
feedback loops and, 33
inflammation, 15–16
list of, 16–17, 33
not having, 9, 18

Tarragon-Lemon Chicken, 222
Teas. See Beverages
Tea tree oil, 52–53
Testing for candida, 34–43
about: overview of, 34–35
blood tests, 37–38
combined testing, 40
cost of tests, 43
deciding to pursue, 34–35
localization of tests, 42
saliva tests, 39–40
sensitivity of tests, 42–43
specificity of tests, 42
Spit Test, 40–41
stool tests, 36–37
trusting the tests, 41–43, 272
urine tests, 38–39
Testing for hydrochloric acid, 83
Thyme, 54
Time, cooking, 106
Time commitment, for diet, 103–4
Tomatillos
Beef Tenderloin in Morita Chili
and Tomatillo Sauce, 260
Red and Green Gazpacho, 183
Salsa Verde, 136
Tomatoes
about: benefits of, 283; making
your own sauce, 117; as
superfood, 283

Chesapeake Stew, 235
Gazpacho, 170
Guacamole Picado, 131
Homemade Ketchup, 204
Red and Green Gazpacho, 183
Roasted Plum Tomatoes, 198
sauces with. See Sauces and
marinades
Tomato and Jicama Guacamole,
128
Tomato-Mint Soup, 142
Tuna Salad with Beefsteak
Tomatoes, 156
Tortilla chip alternative, 183
Toxic chemicals. See Chemicals
Treating candida, 45–63
about: overview of, 45
fatty acids for, 59–61
herbs for. See Herbs and spices
medications for, 46–48
probiotics for. See Probiotics
what not to use, 61–63
Trowbridge, Dr. John, 10
Truss, Dr. Orian, 10, 90
Tuna. See Fish and seafood
Turkey
Hamburger or Ground Turkey
Hash, 255
Mishmash, 247
Turmeric, 291–92
Turpentine, 62
Tuscan Chicken, 221
Tyramine, 94–95, 98, 99

Ulcers
duodenal, 78
esophageal, 78
folic acid (vitamin B_9) and, 81
gastric, 78
H. pylori and, 78
iodine and, 80
iron and, 79–80

medications for, 82–83. See also
Antacids
minerals and, 81–82
nutrient losses and, 78–79
protein and, 79
testing for HCl, 83
ulcers, 78–84
vitamin B_{12} and, 80–81
Undecenoic acid, 20, 60–61
Urine tests, 38–39

Vaginal infections, 279–80
Vegetables. See also specific
vegetables
about: avoiding during candida
diet, 98; candida-fighting
benefits, 98–99, 110; epigenetic
behavior and, 95–96; GMOs,
112–13; included on candida
diet, 98
Mixed Vegetables, 188
soups with. See Soups and stews
Vegetable Curry, 194
Vegetable Stock, 167
Vegetarians and vegans, 275
Virulence, of candida, 21
Vitamin B_9 (folic acid), 81
Vitamin B_{12}, 80–81

Water, drinking, 102–3, 276
Watercress
Fresh Tuna with Watercress
Salad, 155
Hugo's Emerald Mayonnaise, 147
Week 9, adding foods back in, 103,
277, 278–79

Yams. See Sweet potatoes and yams
Yes Foods, 97–103, 275

Zielinski, Dr. Christina, 15–16, 71, 73
Zinc, 82
Zucchini. See Squash